Other Books by Clarence Bass

RIPPED: *The Sensible Way to Achieve Ultimate Muscularity*

RIPPED 2: *The All-new Companion Volume to* RIPPED

RIPPED 3: *The Recipes, the Routines, and the Reasons*

THE LEAN ADVANTAGE: *Four Years of the Ripped Q & A Department*

THE LEAN ADVANTAGE 2: *The Second Four Years*

THE LEAN ADVANTAGE 3: *Four More Years*

LEAN FOR LIFE: *The Lifestyle Approach to Leanness*

CHALLENGE YOURSELF: *Leanness, Fitness & Health*

GREAT EXPECTATIONS: *Health, Fitness, Leanness— Without Suffering*

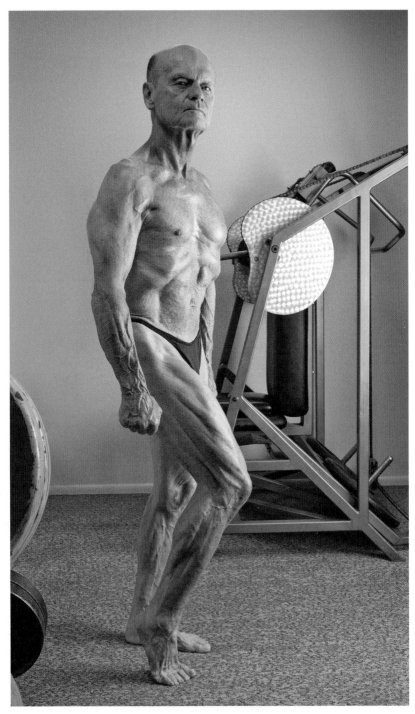

The Author at 75. *(Photo by Laszlo Bencze)*

TAKE CHARGE

Fitness at the Edge of Science

by Clarence Bass

Carol Bass, *Editor*

Clarence Bass' RIPPED™ Enterprises,
Albuquerque, New Mexico
ISBN 978-0-9747682-5-0

To Ralph Carpinelli,
who inspired this book.
He leaves no rock unturned

And to Carole Wright,
whose composition and design magic has
enhanced our books from the beginning

Published by Clarence Bass' Ripped™ Enterprises
P.O. Box 51236
Albuquerque, New Mexico 87181 U.S.A.
505-266-5858 FAX 505-266-9123
E-mail: cncbass@aol.com
Website: www.cbass.com

RIPPED™ is the trademark of Clarence and Carol Bass

Library of Congress Control Number 2012923322
ISBN 978-0-9747682-5-0

Cover design by Randy McMullen, Visual Communications
Albuquerque, New Mexico

Composition and design by Wright Graphics
Nixon, Nevada

Manufactured by Thomson-Shore, Inc.
Dexter, Michigan, U.S.A.

Front cover photo and back cover exercise photos by *Laszlo Bencze*
Physique photo on back cover by *Pat Berrett*

WARNING

Any application of the recommendations in this book is at the reader's sole discretion and risk.

The information in this book is intended for people in good health. If you have medical problems—of any nature—see your doctor before starting a diet or exercise program. Even if you have no known health problems, it is advisable to consult your doctor before making any major changes in your lifestyle.

If you are out of shape or not accustomed to exercise and want to start training, follow the advice of the American Medical Association. "Start slowly and increase the vigor and duration of the activity as your fitness improves." Walking is a good place to start for most people.

Contents

CHAPTER ONE
  Take Charge   **9**

Taking Charge   10
Evolving Goals   11
Aerobics   12
Biomarkers   14
Positive Psychology   17

CHAPTER TWO
  Forget Heavy, Think Effort   **19**

Ralph's Revelation   20
Many Ways   23
Effort Builds Muscle—
  Specificity Principle Prevails   26

CHAPTER THREE
  The Rise Of Intervals   **33**

The Tabata Protocol   34
Half-Minute Sprints Build Endurance!   36
Intervals for (Almost) Everyone   39
Sub-Max Intervals   42

CHAPTER FOUR
  The Aerobic-Strength Alliance   **47**

Strength Training Builds Endurance!   48
Muscle Carries Aerobic Punch   50

Strength Training Builds Muscle—
and Mitochondria 52
Combination Training Works 58
More Bang for the Buck 59

CHAPTER FIVE
Exercise And The Brain   63

Train Your Brain 64
Reboot Your Brain with Exercise 67
Both Aerobics and Weights Boost Brain Power 71
Miracle-Gro for the Brain 74

CHAPTER SIX
Exercise And Aging   81

New Pattern of Aging 82
Live Fit, Live Long 84
Athletes Winning Over Age 86
Exercise Proves Amazing Rejuvenator 90
Exercise Overcome 30 Years of Aging 92
Bending the Aging Curve 94

CHAPTER SEVEN
Too Much Sitting   101

Too Much Sitting Is Risky—
Even for People Who Train 102
Fight Back Against Too Much Sitting 105
Walking Combats Obesity 107
Another Reason to Keep Moving 108
Mother Nature's Recycling and
Vitality Mechanism 112

CHAPTER EIGHT
Fitness & Health   117

Miracle of Movement 118
Strength and Fitness Fight Cancer
Independently 121
The Awesome Power of Exercise—
Help for Schizophrenics 125
Interval Training Reduces Arterial Stiffness 128
Physical Activity Matters, Fitness Matters More 130
Change Your Lifestyle, Change Your Life 134

CHAPTER NINE
Healthy Eating   139

U.S. News & World Report Ranks Diets 140
Cutting Saturated Fat Alone Not Enough 146
How Much Protein Can Muscles Use? 149
Mediterranean-Style Diet Good for
    Brain & Heart 153
Balanced Diet Keeps Weight Off 155

CHAPTER TEN
Dieting Dynamics   159

Weight Loss Is a Dynamic Process—
    Not a Straight Line 160
Managing Food Instincts 165
Exercise Curbs Appetite—
    Our Gut Brain Does the Same 169
It's the Body Fat that Matters 171
Small Calorie Reduction,
    Large Weight Change 174
Hearty Breakfast More Important
    than Calories 176

CHAPTER ELEVEN
Personality Traits   182

The Longevity Project 182
Attitude Matters 188

CHAPTER TWELVE
Take Charge People   193

Truck Driver on the Road to Fitness 196
Businessman Rises to Fitness Challenge 201
Deborah Finds Her Way 203
Law Professor Thrives on Short,
    Efficient Workouts 208
Wayne Gallasch—World Record Holder at 70 213

POSTSCRIPT
My Training Routine, In Brief   219

ACKNOWLEDGMENTS   223

Chapter One

Take Charge

Taking Charge

Bill Pearl, my long time role model and the gold standard in the bodybuilding world, says my strength is that I never stop learning.

Weight training grabbed my attention when I was about 12 —and never let go. I started learning then and added to my knowledge with the passing years. I began with strength training basics and later added new dimensions of fitness one by one: nutrition, aerobic exercise, weight control, motivation, exercise physiology, and health.

This book is about new things I've learned in the last several years—and how they can help readers take charge and improve their lives. The wonders of modern science keep uncovering new ways we can help ourselves live longer, stronger, and healthier.

The paths to success in fitness and health have never been more open and diverse. We can take charge in ways that suit us, ways that we enjoy and do best.

For example, there are many forms of resistance training that build strength and muscle. Some of them also build aerobic capacity. On the other hand, some forms of aerobic exercise also build strength. What's more, both strength training and aerobic exercise improve brain and other bodily functions. Another emerging area is diet dynamics, expanding our understanding

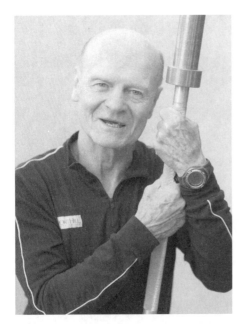

Let's Get Started.
Photo by Laszlo Bencze

of the idiosyncrasies of dieting and weight loss. We'll talk about these and many other new developments—along with a few old ones that have reemerged.

That barely scratches the surface of the wondrous opportunities opening up to people willing to take charge of their bodies and their lives.

Evolving Goals

When I started lifting weights in the fifth grade, my goal was to become an athlete like my dad. I wanted to put on some muscle and get stronger. As the magic of weight training began to work, I upped my sights to becoming as strong as my school chums. Before long I was competing at the high school level, and then the city, state, and regional level. My training was driven by competition. I eventually won national recognition as an Olympic weightlifter and as a bodybuilder. My highest achievements were as a bodybuilder, where I won the overall "Most Muscular Man" award in the Past-40 Mr. USA.

About that time my focus began to change. I began to realize that the only competitor who really counted was me. I had no control over what others did or achieved, but I had complete charge of myself. I could set my sights on any goal that excited me and train in ways I thought best to achieve that goal. I was in charge of myself. I set the rules and judged the results. When I achieved one goal I chose another goal. I looked for ways I could reasonably expect to improve. It worked marvelously well.

As the years rolled by, I became more enthralled with the process, especially for its incredible long-term results. Again, I was competing with myself. I saw people all around me who looked and acted old at 40 and beyond. I decided to follow another path, one that I set for myself.

I gauged what I could do based on my own results. I decided to ignore my age as much as possible. I kept pushing myself to improve in ways that I found realistic and appealing. I set goals based on my own experience, not my age.

When I encountered road blocks, I looked for ways to overcome them, not by force, but by using my mind and methods I have learned in a lifetime of study and taking care of myself. It has almost always worked. At 75, it's still working. I intend to keep training and looking for ways I can improve.

In short, I have done what I hope you will do: take charge.

The process has been amazingly rewarding. The last few years have been filled with new discoveries in the areas I've already touched on, and more. Discoveries that all of us—men and women, young and old—can use to shape our future.

Let's begin with a look back, at two landmark books, one on aerobic exercise and the other on the benefits of strength training. To understand where we're going it helps to know where we've been.

Aerobics

Names and dates are not my strong suit, but I never forget the name *aerobics* and the date 1968. Aerobics is the term coined by Dr. Kenneth H. Cooper to describe a system of exercise that increases oxygen uptake capacity and produces other beneficial changes in the body. The date is the year Cooper's landmark book *Aerobics* was published. Carol and I read the book shortly after it came out and have been doing some form of aerobic exercise ever since. We were part of a growing crowd.

Dr. Cooper's book, along with promotion by Bill Bowerman, Frank Shorter, Dr. George Sheehan, Jim Fixx, and a few others, set off the jogging movement. The number of Americans who jog grew from 100,000 in 1968 to 40 million in 2011.

In the decades after the publication of *Aerobics*, fitness came to mean heart, lung, and circulatory system capability. Fitness and oxygen uptake capacity became essentially synonymous. Fitness meant aerobic fitness. The strength of bones and muscles didn't count for much; they were thought of as largely cosmetic.

"Muscular fitness is of some value, but it is too limited," Cooper wrote in *Aerobics*. "It concentrates on only one system in the body, one of the least important ones, and has limited beneficial effect on the essential organs or overall health. It's like putting a lovely new coat of paint on an automobile that really needs an engine overhaul."

In *Aerobics*, Dr. Cooper introduced a point system for improving oxygen uptake capacity. "Each exercise requires a certain amount of energy, consequently a certain amount of oxygen," he wrote. "This oxygen requirement can be measured, and this is the basis of the point system. Each exercise is assigned a certain number of points, based on the amount of oxygen required to perform it."

Cooper favored exercises that create a significant oxygen re-

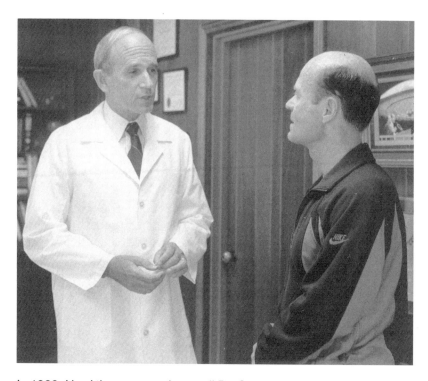

In 1989, I had the opportunity to tell Dr. Cooper how his landmark book made me aware of the importance of aerobic exercise.

Photo by Justin Joseph

quirement, discouraging those with such a low requirement that you'd have to spend hours doing them, or those that build up an oxygen debt too rapidly to have the desired training effect.

"The best exercises are running, swimming, cycling, walking, stationary running, handball, basketball and squash, and in just about that order," he stated. "Isometrics, weight lifting and calisthenics...don't even make the list."

"There is no way I know to lift a strict muscle-producing exercise into an oxygen-demanding activity," he added. Weight lifting doesn't last long enough to have a training effect on the heart, lung, and circulatory system, according to Cooper.

On the other end of the continuum, bowling failed to make his list. It's over too fast, Cooper explained. "Three hours of this may give some physical benefits, but you score a minimum number of points."

Dr. Cooper also frowned on exercises that make you huff and puff, but are over too quickly for a "steady state" to be established. Running or cycling for a short distance or swimming a few laps didn't make the grade for Cooper. "They have no place in an ordinary physical fitness program," he wrote.

Cooper prescribed exercises that "demand oxygen without producing an intolerable oxygen debt, so that they can be continued for long periods."

This steady-state fitness prescription was the standard for decades, and continues to govern the training of many to this day; it may still be the model followed by the majority of fitness-minded individuals.

As we will see, Cooper's original prescription is not the only road to fitness—and may not be the best model for many, perhaps most, people. It's certainly not the most efficient.

That said, Dr. Cooper's seminal book changed the lives of Americans for the better and influenced people all over the world. He continues to be a hugely positive force in preventive medicine and all-around fitness—with 22 additional books to his credit. Importantly, Cooper has moderated his view on weight training; he now tells patients to shift their workouts toward more strength training as they age.

The other landmark book, published 23 years later, began the trend toward parity for aerobic and strength training. A new day was dawning for those of us looking for alternative routes to total fitness.

Biomarkers

BIOMARKERS: The 10 Determinates of Aging You Can Control (Simon and Schuster, 1991) by William J. Evans, PhD, and Irwin H. Rosenberg, MD, professors of nutrition and medicine at Tufts University, changed the landscape of fitness. Strength training began to take its place as an equal partner with aerobics. Moreover, strength training became the senior partner for taking the worry out of aging.

The book featured landmark studies at the USDA Human Nutrition Research Center on Aging (located at Tufts University) showing that people past middle age are able to gain muscle and increase their strength by as much as 200%. More importantly, muscle and strength were found to be the key controllable factors associated with aging.

To paraphrase Satchel Paige, the ageless baseball pitcher, biomarkers are those things that tell how old you would be "if you didn't know how old you was." In *Biomarkers*, Evans and Rosenberg isolated the signposts of vitality that can be altered for the better by changes in lifestyle, leading to more vibrant health for young and old. Here they are in order of importance:

1) Muscle Mass, 2) Strength, 3) Basal Metabolic Rate, 4) Body Fat Percentage, 5) Aerobic Capacity, 6) Blood-sugar Tolerance, 7) Cholesterol/HDL Ratio, 8) Blood Pressure, 9) Bone Density, and 10) Ability to Regulate Internal Temperature

Significantly, all 10 biomarkers can be revived or improved through strength training.

To help people understand how strength training affects the biomarkers, the authors coined the term "sarcopenia" to describe an ailment that affects many people, especially the old, and deprives them of their independence. "Sarco" refers to flesh, "penia" means a reduction in amount. So sarcopenia describes an overall weakening of the body caused by a change in body composition in favor of fat and at the expense of muscle. Unfortunately, sedentary people usually begin losing muscle and gaining fat around the age of 25.

Weight training prevents or reverses sarcopenia; it replaces fat with muscle.

Evans and Rosenberg found that the first biomarker, muscle mass, is responsible for the vitality of your whole physiological apparatus. Muscle mass and strength (the second signpost) are our primary biomarkers. They're the lead dominoes, so to speak. When they start to topple, the other biomarkers soon follow. On the other hand, when muscle mass and strength are maintained, the other indicia are likewise maintained. That is where strength training comes into play. Aerobic exercise and diet are important, but strength training, according to Evans and Rosenberg, is pivotal if you want to stay young longer.

In a 15-year retrospective, *Tufts University Health & Nutrition Letter* (May 2006) found that subsequent research had continued to support the basic premise of *Biomarkers*—that strength training holds the key to successful aging. The *Tufts Letter* highlighted a number of basic points made by Evans and Rosenberg. We'll touch on two here that are often overlooked: the importance of body composition and the effect of strength training on aerobic capacity.

First, the average person may be inclined to focus on losing or maintaining bodyweight. That's not good enough. Your target should be body composition, improving your ratio of muscle to fat. The key is to minimize "biologically inactive" fat tissue and maximize "biologically active" muscle mass. "People with a greater ratio of muscle to fat enjoy a higher metabolism and

15

don't have to worry as much about gaining weight or about how much they eat—[because] that active tissue burns more calories."

The second point is the effect of strength training on the fifth biomarker, aerobic capacity. Aerobic exercise is important, but strength training is central to staying young longer. In point of fact, strength training increases the effectiveness of aerobic exercise. Here's why, as explained in the *Tufts Letter*.

"While both young and older people benefit from regular aerobic exercise—the kind that makes you huff and puff—the positive changes in older people come almost entirely in the muscles' ability to utilize oxygen, rather than in the heart or cardiovascular system."

That's another reason why you need the added muscle mass which comes from strength training. "When you build muscle, you create more muscle cells to consume oxygen. The more demand for oxygen from your muscles, the greater your utilization of oxygen and your aerobic capacity." (We'll elaborate on this often overlooked point in future chapters.)

As noted, fitness and aerobic capacity had become essentially synonymous—but now, with the publication of *Biomarkers*, strength training was adding a new dimension.

Dr. Leonard Schwartz, a 57-year-old Pittsburg psychiatrist, made this point (before the publication of *Biomarkers*) in his

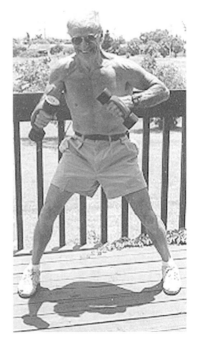

Len Schwartz was a free thinker, ahead of his time in many ways. He used the *Heavyhands* he invented with gusto—to build fitness and muscle.
Photo provided by Dr. Schwartz before his passing in 2010 at the age of 84.

book *Heavyhands, The Ultimate Exercise*, published in 1982. Schwartz recommended the use of light dumbbells for high repetitions to develop overall fitness. His own guinea pig, Schwartz developed both muscle and aerobic fitness. In so doing, he was perhaps the first to recognize the value of weight lifting in building aerobic capacity.

* * *

Having snapshots of the supposed polar opposites on the exercise spectrum, aerobic exercise on one end and strength training on the other, let's turn to psychology for help deciding where to position yourself for maximum training results and satisfaction. As a take charge trainer, you'll want to do that in a way that suits you best. In the next section we'll tell you about a new way to decide, the psychologically sound way.

Positive Psychology

Enjoyment is the key to long-term success in training. Almost no one will stay on a diet they don't enjoy. The same goes for exercise. Feeling good about your training makes all the difference in the world. People who enjoy their training are far more likely to stick with it than those who force themselves to train in a prescribed way. I knew early on that I liked lifting weights. I was built for lifting; I wasn't cut out to run marathons. I found my sport and stuck with it.

"I do not believe that you should devote overly much effort to correcting your weaknesses," Martin E. P. Seligman, PhD, father of the positive psychology movement, wrote in *Authentic Happiness* (Free Press, 2002). "Rather, I believe that the highest success in living and the deepest emotional satisfaction comes from building and using your signature strengths."

That doesn't mean you have to be a champion; it simply means you'll do better in an activity that you find satisfying. Satisfaction, for most people, comes from making progress, being successful in the competition with yourself. Picking your own field of play substantially improves your odds. My own situation provides an example.

Muscle heads do best when they choose activities with a strength element. For example, when I pursue competitive rowing, a largely aerobic activity, I focus on the 500 meter distance (basically a sprint) rather than the standard 2000 meters. On the other hand, marathon types will probably be well advised to pick events with an endurance component; the 5,000 meter row might be a good choice. People in the middle, the majority, will probably do best with the standard 2000 meter distance.

Another option might be to choose an exercise mode that incorporates both strength and endurance. Heavyhands is an example; it bridges the gap between aerobic and strength training.

There is no "best way" to train, there are many. Finding and pursuing ways that suit your body and personality is what taking charge is about. New discoveries are uncovering more information and more options. More options mean better odds of success for everyone, pros, amateurs, men, women, young or old.

* * *

In the next chapter, we'll begin talking about new research findings from scientists far and wide—Germany, Japan, England, Sweden, Norway, Canada, Brazil, from coast to coast in the USA, and more—and the practical and exciting ways their discoveries can be used to help you reach your goals. We'll start with a breakthrough in strength training.

Chapter Two

Forget Heavy, Think Effort

Ralph's Revelation

An eye-opening event in Ralph Carpinelli's basement changed his thinking on heavy lifting: "My friend Roman was the only one I knew who never cared about his one-rep maximum for any exercise. One day in my basement I convinced him to try a maximum single in the bench press. At 140 pounds body weight, he bench pressed 300 pounds relatively easily and said: *That's enough; I don't want to hurt myself.* That was when I first realized that you could get very strong and build muscle without ever having to lift very heavy weights."

Fortunately, Dr. Ralph N. Carpinelli was well positioned to test the validity of the lightning-bolt revelation that struck in his basement home gym. He teaches exercise physiology at Adelphi University in Garden City, New York. From his perch in Adelphi's Human Performance Laboratory he made an exhaustive review of the scientific literature and, in 2008, reported his findings in the *Journal of Exercise Science and Fitness.*

Many people, including those who need it most, are turned off by weight training. They imagine themselves having to lift heavy weights. Carpinelli's report has the potential to change that perception—and get many more people pumping iron.

Dr. Carpinelli's review led him to conclude that effort, not heavy weights, is the key factor in building muscle and strength. That breakthrough finding made resistance training suitable for just about anyone. It gave people many more strength training options.

Ralph's conclusion was news to many lifters, including me. "Only the heaviest possible weight will bring the maximum number of muscle fibers into action," I wrote in my book *Ripped 2.* The underlying idea is correct—but there's more to the story. Most experts in the field have made the same error.

Carpinelli's analysis is based on the *size principle*, which governs the manner in which muscle fibers are activated. The size principle is "perhaps the most supported principle in neurophysiology," Carpinelli states. So let's start there. What is it?

The size principle is a law that explains the order in which muscle fibers contract. In a nut shell, it says small fibers contract before large fibers.

The small fibers are slow-twitch, and the large fibers are fast-twitch. The slow-twitch fibers are the endurance fibers, which predominate in marathon runners and other endurance athletes. Like the Energizer Bunny, they don't give out, they keep on contracting. They don't generate much force, however. Fast-twitch fibers are the strength fibers, which rule the roost in sprinters, weight lifters, and other strength athletes. They are strong, but fatigue rapidly. Most of us are born with a roughly equal balance of slow/small and fast/large fibers.

The bottom line is that it's much harder to turn on fast fibers than it is slow fibers; it takes more current or stimulus, more intensity—more effort. Importantly, muscle fibers contract for all they're worth, or not at all. Muscle fibers are either on or off; there is no in-between. This is called the "all or none" law of muscle fiber contraction. Fibers that aren't stimulated don't contract and grow stronger. They eventually wither and die.

Okay then, here's the pertinent question: Do heavy loads stimulate more fibers? Not necessarily, says Carpinelli.

So, you may ask, how does he know? How do scientists decide such questions?

The most objective way is with activation level (AL) studies, which measure muscle fiber response. AL studies compare voluntary (human) and electrically induced response. If the voluntary response matches the electrical response, AL is 100%. If the voluntary response is less, the shortfall will be expressed as a percentage of the induced response.

Dr. Carpinelli looked to the "most relevant...activation level (AL) study with the greatest practical application to resistance training."

In the study, researchers compared voluntary and induced muscle fiber recruitment after 5 RM, 10 RM and 20 RM dumbbell curls. (RM stands for *repetition maximum*) They reported no significant difference in voluntary motor unit AL after 5 RM (95.5%), 10 RM (93.5%), and 20 RM (95.1%).

Their clear-cut conclusion: "The commonly repeated suggestion that maximal strength methods (resistance heavier than a 6 RM) produce greater neural adaptations or increases in neural drive was not substantiated in this study."

"In fact," Carpinelli emphasized, "their study unequivocally demonstrates the direct relationship between intensity of effort—not the amount of resistance—and voluntary motor unit activation."

Dr. Carpinelli also reviewed studies that measured strength gains using different reps and resistance. He found only one study that reported some strength advantages for low reps and heavy resistance; the finding was, however, inconclusive.

The authors in that study concluded: "It has often been accepted that improved strength/power results from high intensity/low volume training, whereas low intensity/high volume training maximizes muscle hypertrophy. Based on data from the present investigation, this *may not be entirely true*. Indeed, data from the present investigation suggest low and intermediate RM training induces similar muscular adaptations, at least after short-term training in previously untrained subjects." (Emphasis mine)

Perhaps it should come as no surprise that proponents of heavier-is-better training do not cite this study.

Carpinelli found many studies showing no advantage for heavier-is-better training. He listed 20 resistance training studies that reported no significant difference in strength gains for 2 reps to 20 reps lifted to failure (RM).

Carpinelli singled out a study of 10 pairs of identical twins as especially "noteworthy." Identical twins are ideal subjects for study because they have the same genetic make-up. They take the "nature" out of the "nature-or-nurture" question. They lay bare the difference between training protocols. If heavier is better, comparison of identical twins should show it.

The study found "no significant difference in the strength gain as a result of training with 7-10 RM (13.2%), or 15-20 RM (12.8%)."

Listen to Dr. Carpinelli's bottom line; it's liberating.

Resistance is largely a matter of "personal preference," wrote Carpinelli. "If a maximal—or near maximal—effort is applied at the end of a set of repetitions, the evidence strongly suggests that the different external forces produced with different amounts of resistance elicit similar outcomes."

That's it. So simple, yet so meaningful—and potentially influential.

"If the size principle was correctly applied, effective resistance training may appeal to a larger proportion of the population," Carpinelli continued. "This would include competitive and recreational athletes as well as those in the general population who perceive resistance exercise as the lifting of very heavy weights and therefore potentially dangerous." He continued, "Because some people may have a fear of injury—that need not exist—the heavier-is-better perception may actually be a deterrent to resistance training, which deprives those most in need of health-related benefits."

* * *

If ever there was a landmark review study in the resistance

training field, this is it. Dr. Carpinelli's impressive—and bold—effort has the potential to open the door to the health and fitness benefits of resistance training for millions of additional people.

The take-away message: If you enjoy lifting heavy, go for it. If you'd prefer to work with lighter weight and more reps, that's fine too. Either way, heavy or light, the key to progress is effort on the last few reps. The choice is yours.

*   *   *

In the next section, we'll tell you about a study that reviews some of the many options to which Carpinelli's breakthrough finding has opened the door. It will stagger—and stimulate—your imagination.

Many Ways

Effort comes in many forms—and scientists are counting the ways.

Sandee Jungblut, an associate of Dr. Carpinelli at the Adelphi University Human Performance Laboratory, combed the literature for practical applications of effort-based training and reported her findings in the journal *Medicina Sportiva* the year after Carpinelli's landmark review.

Again examining AL studies, Jungblut found, like Carpinelli, that the choice is yours. You can lift heavy or light, low reps, mid-range reps, or high reps. Your muscles will respond the same—as long as the last rep or two challenges your level of strength.

Think about that. Your options are very wide indeed. Any rep range from 5 to 20 will stimulate your muscles to grow stronger.

As wide ranging as that sounds, Jungblut expanded the review, finding still more studies.

She moved on to two noteworthy studies using strength and muscle gain as a measure of effectiveness. The studies provide still more options.

The first study compared fast and slow reps, time under load (TUL) to be precise. The end points were strength gain and increase in muscle thickness. One group performed relatively fast reps (1s positive and 1s negative), and the other group did slower reps (3s up and 3s down).

Both groups significantly increased strength and muscle thickness. There was no significant difference in results between groups.

Jungblut commented: "The large difference in the amount of

resistance used [and TUL] for training did not produce a significant difference in strength gains or muscle thickness between
the training groups, because the effort at the end of each set
was similar [maximal]."

Fast and slow reps are equally effective. Again, the choice is
yours; you can lift fast or slow. If you lift slowly you won't have
to use as much weight; that's because you take the momentum
out of the lift.

The second resistance training study will probably surprise
you, as it did me. It compared traditional weight resistance
training (WRT) and manual resistance training (MRT).

I'm going to give almost all of the details so you'll understand
the significance of this study. The results suggest that resis-
tance-training options are almost limitless. It appears that any
form of resistance that requires maximum or near maximum
effort will build strength and muscle.

Healthy college students (male and female) were assigned
to either a traditional weight training group (WRT) or a manual resistance group (MRT). The amount of resistance can't
be quantified with MRT, because the resistance is "provided
manually by another person (a spotter)" rather than by bar-
bells, dumbbells, or machines. "By targeting comparable muscle
groups and exercise movements as closely as possible" the MRT
exercises were similar to the WRT exercises.

Free weight bench press and squat exercises were used to
measure strength gain in both groups. The authors of the study
noted: "The regular training group had an apparent advantage
in the free weight...testing because the same equipment was
used for training and assessment, whereas the manual training
group did not use any free weights or exercise machines during
the 14 week program."

Nevertheless, both groups showed similar and significant increases in muscular strength for both the bench press and the
squat.

Jungblut explained how that could happen: "[While] the
amount of resistance applied by the spotters...was not known in
the MRT group...the stimulus for similar strength gains in both
groups was most likely the same degree of effort—maximal."

There's more, but you get the idea loud and clear. The over-
whelming weight of the evidence (82 out of 90 studies) is that
any mode of resistance training that elicits a high degree of effort builds strength.

This concept may have been misunderstood—or ignored—in

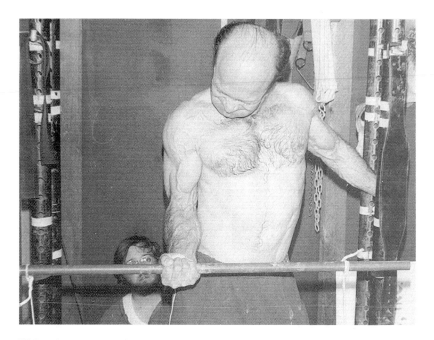

This photo, taken in 1974 by my neighbor Bill Vollendorf, shows me resisting the pull of an electrical motor. The effect on the muscle was immense—but there was a problem. The motor always won. My training partner (controlling the motor in the background) and I eventually lost interest, because we never knew whether we were making progress. MRT would present the same problem.

recent times, but it is not new. Jungblut says it has been known for many years that effort is the key to strength gains.

"A half century ago in [*Science* 1957]," she wrote, "Henneman... explained that increasingly larger motor units require progressively greater increases in the intensity of the stimulus." Greater intensity, not poundage, makes muscles grow stronger.

What's more, Jungblut related that Digby G. Sale, PhD, published a lengthy review on the practical application of resistance training in *Exercise Sport Science Review* (1987) explaining that "the trainee may execute a single maximum repetition; or... perform repetitions to muscular fatigue with five repetitions or 10 repetitions." Importantly, Sale further observed "that motor unit activation would not be maximal at the beginning of the 5 RM or 10 RM sets but would be maximal at the termination of either set and similar to the 1 RM motor unit activation.

* * *

More recently, the substance of the Carpinelli and Jungblut

review studies has been borne out on both sides of the Atlantic, by controlled trial at McMaster University in Canada (Burd, PLoS, 2010) and literature review in the UK (Fisher, *Medicina Sportiva*, 2011).

My long-time friend Richard Winett, Professor of Psychology at Virginia Tech and an astute trainer, described these recent developments in cosmic terms: "In some ways, these findings on resistance training...are the equivalent of saying the earth isn't actually flat; it's round. The way we looked at things before has now been turned upside down."

* * *

A U-turn such as this is understandably slow to be accepted; some just don't buy it. Fortunately, we have an impressive new study from McMaster University confirming earlier findings on load and muscle building—and carving out a narrow qualification that may speed acceptance of the new training model.

Effort Builds Muscle— Specificity Principle Prevails

"Perhaps the most interesting finding from our work is that hypertrophy in the [heavy] and [light] conditions was equivalent..., [but training load] did have a clear impact on...strength gains," Cameron J. Mitchell, Stuart Phillips et al wrote in the *Journal of Applied Physiology* (April 2012).

This training study from McMaster University confirmed their earlier finding that light weights are just as effective for building muscle as heavy weights; the critical factor is the effort put into each set.

In an important new finding, their data hewed to the long-established specificity principle when it came to strength gains; to lift heavy weights you must lift heavy weights. Finally, their results also suggested that additional volume—more sets—may build more muscle.

A distinguishing feature of the new study is its 10 week timespan. Their two earlier studies tested the effect of a single bout of training. One study (Burd, PLoS, August 9, 2010) compared the effect of training to failure with 30% and 80% of 1RM, while the second study (Burd, *Journal of Physiology*, August 15, 2010) compared training to failure with 70% of 1RM for 1 set and 3 sets. The first study found no difference in the resulting muscle

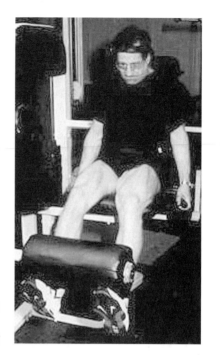

Professor Winett knows a lot about heavy weights—and effort.
Photo courtesy of Winett

building, while the second study found that 3 sets builds more muscle than 1 set.

The new study tested the effect of training to failure three times a week under three training conditions: 1) One set at 80% of maximum load, 2) Three sets at 80% of maximum, and 3) Three sets at 30% of maximum.

The test exercise was the unilateral knee extension, which works the front part of the upper limb (quadriceps). Changes in muscle size were measured by magnetic resonance imaging (MRI) and strength by increases in one-rep maximum (1RM).

All three training conditions produced significant increases in quadriceps volume. The heavy and light groups doing 3 sets gained essentially the same: 30% load produced an increase of 6.8%, and 80% produced a gain of 7.2%. The group doing a single set to failure with 80%, however, showed a gain of only 3.2%, about half as much as the groups doing 3 sets.

Strength gains were more tightly bunched. All three training conditions produced significant increases in 1RM strength, but the increase was a bit greater in the groups lifting 80% for 1 and 3 sets. The difference in strength gain was small, but undeniable.

What do these findings mean? What's the explanation?

First and foremost, the 10-week training study confirms the

principal finding of the earlier single bout studies by the same group—and the results of Dr. Carpinelli's review study. For muscle building, it makes no difference whether the weight used is heavy or light. The choice is yours. Professor Stuart Phillips summed it up for Science Daily (April 30, 2012): "Our study provides evidence for a simpler paradigm, where a much broader range of loads including quite light loads can induce muscle growth, provided it is lifted to the point where it is difficult to maintain good form."

The departure came in building strength, where heavy weights provided a slight but clear advantage. The long-established specificity principle asserted its primacy. "These data confirm the specificity principle of training in regards to muscle strength and endurance," Cameron-Phillips and colleagues wrote in summarizing their findings.

"These results suggest that practice with a heavy relative load is necessary to maximize gain in 1RM strength," the researchers wrote. "These observations are in line with previous work which has shown that strength gains are specific to the movement that is trained and strength gains are due to a combination of muscle hypertrophy and neural [nerve impulse] adaptations," they continued. "However, it appears that neural adaptations are largely specific to the movement and load used in training."

That makes sense. Lifting an 80% load requires a more dynamic nerve impulse than lifting a 30% load, especially on the early reps. That explains why Olympic weightlifters, who must marshal the maximum possible number of muscle fibers for one Herculean effort, often spend the lion's share of their training time doing single lifts.

On the other hand, an endurance athlete would probably be well advised to lift lighter weights for more repetitions. Notably, the 30% load group in the new study recorded a 30% increase in type 1 endurance fibers compared to only 18% in type 2 strength fibers. Interestingly, the group lifting 80% for 3 sets produced a balanced increase in endurance and strength fibers, 17% and 16%, respectively.

For the vast majority of people—who aren't concerned with how much weight they can lift one time—the thing to remember is that both light and heavy weights produce significant gains in muscle size and strength. "These data show that hypertrophy [muscle size] is generally beneficial to all strength and power tests...," the Cameron-Phillips team wrote. Muscle drives func-

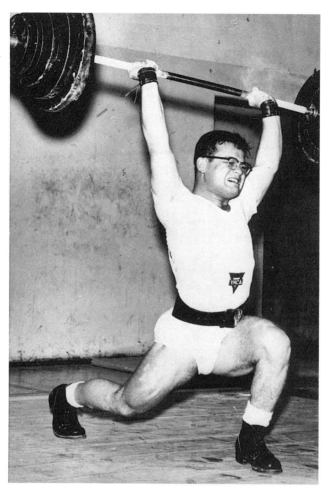

A lift such as the Clean & Jerk, shown here, takes practice with heavy weights. I was one of the youngest lifters in the country to officially Clean & Jerk 300 pounds. I did it in February of 1956, a few months past my 18th birthday, weighing 165. *Photographer unknown*

tionality; it helps you stand up, walk, run, jump, and do the things necessary to live a full and independent life.

Finally, we have the conundrum of sets and muscle size. As noted, the group doing one set showed only half the increase in muscle size seen by the groups doing three sets. Their earlier study produced a similar result—and called for a training study "to delineate the superiority of 1 set or 3 sets for inducing hypertrophy."

We now have the training study, but the jury is still out. Unfortunately, the difference between the 1-set and 3-set groups was not significant. "Interestingly, there was no statistical difference in the degree of quadriceps hypertrophy between the 80%-1 and 80%-3 conditions, despite a mean gain...of ~7% in the 80%-3 condition and only ~3% in the 80%-1 condition," the researchers wrote. "It appears that longer-term training studies may be required to manifest these differences more clearly."

The statistical problem apparently arises out of "the inherent variability in individual response to resistance training," the researchers related. "In fact, when subjects are stratified as high and low responders, 20-25% of subjects exhibit very limited hypertrophic response whereas the top 20-25% show robust muscle hypertrophy that is four to five times greater than that seen in low responders."

Cameron-Phillips and colleagues cautiously concluded: "The results from our study...*suggest* that additional training volume in the form of more sets *may* result in greater muscle hypertrophy." (Emphasis mine)

Unfortunately, that may be as good as it's going to get on the sets issue. It may come down to a matter of personal preference.

Importantly, Cameron-Phillips et al are clear on the main finding: "A lower load lifted to failure resulted in similar hypertrophy as a heavy load lifted to failure."

*   *   *

The problem with doing multiple sets, as I see it, is focus. It's difficult to maintain quality—or intensity—and do many sets. While that's not likely to be a problem in a research setting with a technician overseeing every rep, it is a problem in actual practice. When you plan to do multiple work sets, consciously or unconsciously, you pace yourself; you hold back on the early sets, saving energy for the sets to follow. Like a long-distance runner, you husband your strength. The end result is that some muscle fibers go unused.

On the other hand, do only one work set and you can focus totally on that set without thinking about the sets to come. You are free to make an all-out effort; you don't have to hold anything in reserve. As in a 100-yard dash, you give it all you've got from start to finish. The result is a more intense set, which brings more muscle fibers into action.

Nevertheless, I know that many readers will want to try doing three (or more) sets—as I do from time to time. The difference is that I change the movement or the load on each set; I rarely do the same thing twice. That keeps the challenge fresh and the effort intense. I'll give two examples. (I do one or more warm-up sets before the work set or sets.)

On the leg press, I do the heaviest set first, and then one or two drop-back sets. (I rest between sets.) The top weight wakes up muscle fibers that go unused in the warm-up sets, producing an enhanced response on the drop-back set or sets. For example, I might do 12 reps with 500, 20 with 450, and 25 with 400. The response is staggering; I can barely walk afterward.

Secondly, I do one all-out set with three different exercises for the same body part. For example, for the upper back I do the Nautilus pullover, the lat pulldown, and the dumbbell bent row. This is my normal workout pattern for most body parts; it works especially well for the upper back and chest.

* * *

After reviewing this chapter, Dr. Carpinelli told me in a personal communication that he does not agree that practice with a heavy relative load is necessary to maximize gain in 1RM

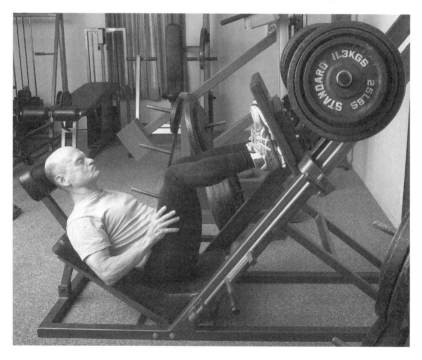

The leg press is a good back-friendly lower body exercise. Unlike the squat, you can focus on effort without worrying about balance. Note how I keep my hands on my thighs to help if I have trouble getting the weight up; I've never failed to get the weight up with my legs, but it's better to be safe than sorry. *Photo by Laszlo Bencze*

strength; he referred me to his review article published June 15, 2011, in the journal *Medicina Sportiva*.

"The only trainees that need to know their 1RM for any exercise are competitive weightlifters and Powerlifters—and they know their 1RM when they practice their sport," he told me, repeating what he wrote in his review article.

"The bottom line to stimulate strength gains is to select a load that requires a reasonable effort on the final repetition of a set and gradually increase the resistance...," Carpinelli wrote. There is little, if any, difference, Carpinelli observed, between a one rep maximum and the final rep of a set done with maximum effort.

If you wait for exercise physiologists to agree on this technical point, you're likely to be waiting a very long time. If you don't plan to compete, forget 1RM and concentrate on improving your performance with submaximal poundages. Select a rep range and manner of performance that suits you and work on improving over time.

Let the researchers duke it out. It makes little or no difference to the vast majority of trainees. Do what suits you.

*   *   *

It's a new day in resistance training. Don't be left behind. Choose any form of resistance training that appeals to you. Heavy, light, one set or many; they all make us stronger and fitter.

Experiment. Find what suits you best—what you enjoy. Take Charge.

*   *   *

In the next chapter we move to the other side of the exercise spectrum and talk about aerobic conditioning. How much, how far, how fast? The "how" questions are being looked at by scientists and research is opening up new ways to think about training. You have options!

Chapter Three
The Rise of Intervals

The Tabata Protocol

Everyone is talking about it today, but that wasn't the case in 1997 when Richard Winett and I began discussing it. Winett, a researcher and lifetime strength and fitness trainer, had been in contact with Dr. Izumi Tabata in Japan. Dr. Tabata was surprised that a middle-aged professor would be interested in trying his aerobic training protocol. He warned Dick that elite speed-skaters were flat on their backs gasping for breath after completing his four-minute regimen.

"What's the most efficient work-rest ratio to improve the cardiovascular system?" Professor Joseph F. Signorile asked in his book *Bending the Aging Curve* (We'll discuss it in Chapter 6). His answer: "The winner is...the old 2:1 standby composed of 20 seconds of work and 10 seconds of recovery."

That describes the Tabata protocol: go all-out for 20 seconds, easy for 10 seconds, and repeat 6 to 8 times. It takes about four minutes—and is amazingly effective. It is also brutal.

"The rate of increase in VO2max is one of the highest ever reported," Tabata wrote in the journal *Medicine and Science in Sports and Exercise* in 1996.

That was exciting. The prospect of rapidly increasing the body's ability to process oxygen (VO2max) and improve performance made fitness-minded people take notice. It didn't happen over night, but people were interested. Up to that time, interval training was thought to be for athletes only. Intervals were notoriously hard; no one thought the public would be interested.

I began writing about a form of intervals—I called them bursts—for bodybuilders in 1986, in my book *Ripped 3*. Not many paid attention, however. Most bodybuilders and others continued doing steady-state aerobics, as recommended by Dr. Ken Cooper and others.

So what did Dr. Tabata's research reveal that changed things?

Tabata compared the effect of moderate-intensity endurance training and his high-intensity interval training protocol on VO2max and anaerobic capacity. Tabata's interval protocol was unique among aerobic training programs for its intensity and brevity. The elapsed time of the moderate-intensity and the high-intensity protocol was drastically different: one hour compared to about four minutes!

Think of that! Total exercise time each week was five hours for the moderate-intensity protocol and about 20 minutes for the high-intensity protocol.

The moderate-intensity protocol will sound familiar; it's the same steady-state aerobic training done by most fitness enthusiasts—then and now.

Both groups exercised on stationary bicycles 5 days a week for 6 weeks. The moderate-intensity group (physically active students) pedaled at 70% of VO2max for 60 minutes. The second group of students did the Tabata protocol: seven to eight sets of 20 seconds at 170% of VO2max, with a 10 second rest period between each bout. Aerobic capacity (VO2max) and anaerobic capacity were continually monitored for both groups. Note again—one group exercised for 60 minutes a day and the other for about four minutes.

In some respects the results were not a surprise, but in others they were earth shaking. The moderate-intensity endurance training program produced a significant increase in VO2max (about 10%), but had no effect on anaerobic (without oxygen) capacity. The high-intensity interval protocol improved VO2max by about 14%, while anaerobic capacity increased by a whopping 28%.

You may ask, What's the advantage of increasing anaerobic capacity? Simply put, it means you can exercise hard longer.

Tabata and his colleagues believed this was the first study to demonstrate an increase in both aerobic and anaerobic power, with and without oxygen. What's more, in an e-mail response to Richard Winett, Tabata wrote, "The fact is that the rate of increase in VO2max [14% for the high-intensity protocol, in only 6 weeks] is one of the highest ever reported in exercise science."

The intensity in the steady state protocol (70% of VO2max)

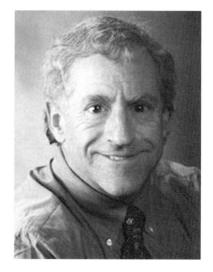

Richard Winett, PhD, a professor of psychology at Virginia Tech, was one of the first (perhaps the first) fitness trainers to show an interest in the brutally hard Tabata Protocol. Dr. Tabata was surprised that a middle-aged professor would be interested in doing his interval training protocol.
Photo courtesy of Winett

did not create an oxygen debt—that's why it's called steady state or pay as you go—so it was predictable that anaerobic capacity would be unchanged. On the other hand, the subjects in the high-intensity interval group exercised to exhaustion; peak blood lactate levels indicated that anaerobic metabolism was being taxed to the max. Therefore, it was not a big surprise that anaerobic capacity increased quite significantly (28%).

What was a surprise, however, is that a 4-minute training program of very-hard 20 second repeats, in the words of the researchers, "may be optimal with respect to improving both the aerobic and the anaerobic energy release systems." That was truly stunning!

The problem with the Tabata protocol was—and is—that few can continue doing it. It takes a streak of masochism to want to do it for very long. It's just too darn hard. It is not fun. That's a major problem for health professionals trying to persuade people to exercise—with little success.

Predictably, they began looking for interval training plans suitable for more people. That started a trend that's still ongoing. It took a while, but it's working. People are starting to pay attention. They get the advantages. They're actually beginning to like intervals.

A big first step to making intervals more acceptable to ordinary trainers came from McMaster University (Hamilton, Ontario, Canada), a hot bed of cutting-edge exercise science. They made the work-rest ratio considerably more user friendly—with outstanding results.

That's what most people are looking for—something that fits their level of fitness and psychological commitment, while achieving their goals.

Half-Minute Sprints Build Endurance!

In marked contrast to Tabata's regimen, the McMaster recovery interval was much longer than the work interval. The results, however, were no less remarkable.

The test group did four to seven "all-out" 30-second sprints on an exercise bicycle with *four-minute rest periods*, six times over two weeks.

Endurance capacity doubled!

"This has the potential to change the way we think about

keeping fit," McMaster University Professor Martin J. Gibala, the lead spokesperson for the new study, told the *London Telegraph* in 2005. "We thought there would be benefits but we did not expect them to be this obvious. It shows how effective short intense exercise can be."

Kirsten Burgomaster and her McMaster colleagues published their results with sprint intervals in the *Journal of Applied Physiology* (June 2005).

Sixteen active students were divided into two groups: half performed two weeks of sprint intervals, and the other half did no training.

"Most strikingly," the Burgomaster team wrote, "cycle endurance capacity increased by 100% after [sprint interval training]." The time to fatigue cycling at about 80% of VO2max increased on average from 26 minutes to 51 minutes! Again, endurance capacity doubled. (As expected, the control group showed no change.)

"To our knowledge, this is the first study to show that sprint training dramatically improves endurance capacity...," the researchers reported. Impressively, the short period of very intense exercise produced improvements "comparable to or higher than previously reported aerobic-based training studies of similar duration."

A few minutes of very intense exercise (12 to 21 minutes over 2 weeks) produced the same or better results than previously shown after two hours a day, five days a week at about 65% of VO2max, or 20 hours over two weeks.

The McMaster study created quite a stir. Professor Gibala was quoted widely in this country, Canada, and in the UK:

"The whole excuse that 'I don't have enough time to exercise' is directly challenged by these findings," Gibala told the *London Telegraph.*

"This type of training is very demanding and requires a high level of motivation; however, less frequent, high intensity exercise can indeed lead to improvements in health and fitness," Gibala told CNN.

"We think there might be a public health message that you can perform intense exercise, but less volume, and obtain similar benefits," Gibala told Canada TV.

The Journal of Applied Physiology found the new study noteworthy enough to merit a thought provoking "Invited Editorial" by Edward F. Coyle, Department of Kinesiology and Health Education, University of Texas at Austin.

Coyle wrote, "[It] serves as a dramatic reminder of the potency" of intense exercise to improve performance, with "implications for improving health." It shows that sprints are "very time efficient, with much bang for the buck."

Researchers are finding that doing long, slow distance training to improve performance is not smart, time-efficient training.

It seems logical, Coyle observed, that "aerobic endurance performance is only enhanced by aerobic endurance training, but it has been proven wrong in the realm of athletics as well as muscle biochemistry."

Coyle observed that middle-distance runners typically include sprint intervals in their training to improve aerobic endurance. "Indeed," he wrote, "it is likely that if an experienced runner or bicyclist had only 2 weeks and very limited time to prepare for a race of [about] 30-minutes...that sprint interval training would become a mainstay of their preparation."

Roger Bannister's preparation to run the first 4-minute mile is a classic case in point. Bannister's workouts were almost exclusively 400-meter sprints with two or three minute recovery between repeats; see *The Perfect Mile*, Houghton Mifflin Company, 2004.

We've learned that interval training dramatically improves endurance. But what accounts for the surprising effectiveness? Very hard 30-second sprints work, but why? What's the precise mechanism? The explanation offered by Professor Coyle is direct and to the point.

Coyle says that the muscle fibers affected in sprint intervals and in steady state exercise are different. "All-out sprint training especially stresses...fast twitch muscle fibers that are remarkably and equally responsive as slow twitch muscle fibers in their ability to increase mitochondrial enzyme activity [oxygen-processing activity]," Coyle explained. "In fact, the low-intensity aerobic exercise that is typically prescribed for endurance training or health is not very effective at increasing aerobic activity in [fast twitch] muscle fibers, which comprise approximately one-half of the fibers within the muscles of most people," he continued. "Thus low-intensity aerobic training is not a very effective or efficient method for maximizing aerobic adaptation in skeletal muscle because it generally does not recruit [fast twitch] fibers."

That's it. No amount of low-intensity aerobic exercise will increase aerobic power—the rate at which oxygen can be used—like sprint interval training.

Simply put, sprint interval training increases the endurance capacity in all muscle fibers, fast and slow, while long slow training leaves half of the fibers unused and untrained. It's like pulling a wagon with one horse, when two would get you a lot farther down the road.

As shown by the Burgomaster study, training the slow and fast fibers with short, hard intervals takes you twice as far.

There is no free lunch, however. Even with four minutes of recovery, high-intensity intervals are taxing. "[Repeated all-out sprints] cause a feeling of severe fatigue lasting for at least 10-20 minutes," Professor Coyle warned. "That is the price for its effectiveness and remarkable time efficiency. It remains to be determined which population, depending on age, health status, and psychology, are most likely to adhere and benefit from sprint interval training."

In summary, Dr. Tabata's research was a stimulus for aerobic trainers to think about the volume and intensity of their training. Later research reinforced this thinking and showed that remarkable results could be obtained in less onerous ways.

* * *

The health status issue of potential interval trainers was soon to be addressed by other researchers.

It was a given that *high-volume* endurance training improves blood flow to the heart and muscles. Are *high-intensity* intervals equally effective, or perhaps more effective? Are intervals safe for people with health issues? Norwegian and Canadian researchers stepped up with additional research.

Canada's McMaster University was, once again, in the vanguard. Intervals, it turns out, are good—often better—for people with heart and other ailments.

Intervals for (Almost) Everyone

Following up on the 2005 Burgomaster findings (discussed above), McMaster University researchers reported in the *American Journal of Physiology* (2008) that "low-volume sprint interval training" produced cardiovascular results similar to high-volume endurance training, with less than half the training time.

Their interval group did four to six 30 second "all-out" stationary-bike sprints, with 4.5 minutes recovery, 3 days a week; the endurance group did 40-60 minutes of moderate-intensity cycling 5 days a week.

Both forms of training improved artery structure and flexibility, and both improved blood flow in the legs.

The study demonstrated that people who are pressed for time can still derive cardiovascular benefits from exercise, Maureen MacDonald, an associate professor of Kinesiology, related in a McMaster University press release. MacDonald, however, specified that they must be willing to work hard for brief periods of time. (We'll come back to the motivation issue in the next section.)

"More and more, professional organizations are recommending interval training during rehabilitation from diseases like chronic [lung] and...cardiovascular disease," MacDonald reported. "We wouldn't be surprised to see more rehabilitation programs adopt this method of training since it is often better tolerated in diseased populations."

Confirming MacDonald's report and prediction, Norwegian researchers reported remarkable results in rehab. We'll look at two studies which make a powerful case for intervals—regardless of age or health status. The McMaster study showed that intervals are on par with continuous exercise for improving health status. The Norwegian studies suggest that intervals are better—and not just because they take less time.

The Norwegians conducted a comparison study like the McMaster study, but with older patients (average age 75) diagnosed with chronic heart failure; they also measured a wider range of cardiovascular and quality of life effects. (*Circulation,* June 4, 2007)

The results were, to say the least, noteworthy—favoring intervals in virtually every respect.

Peak aerobic capacity (VO2max) increased more with intervals than with continuous training; the difference was a jaw-dropping + 46% versus + 14%. The improvement was coupled with a significant beneficial remodeling of the left ventricle (LV), the large chamber of the heart, but only in the interval group. LV ejection fraction, an index of heart function, increased 35% in the interval group, while no improvement was seen in the continuous training group. In addition, pro-brain natriuretic peptide, a marker of the severity of heart failure, declined by 40%–again in the interval group only.

And there's more. As in the McMaster study, artery flexibility and blood flow improved, this time in the principal artery in the upper arm—with "greater improvement" shown by the interval group than the continuous training group.

Quality of life improved in both groups, but again "more

markedly in the interval subjects, which suggests that more intensive physical training is more rewarding," the researchers wrote in their report. "Informal comments from the patients" indicated that the interval group enjoyed the "varied procedure" and that the endurance group found it "quite boring" to walk continuously during the entire exercise period.

Perhaps most surprising was the age and health status of the subjects. "Of particular interest is the old age of the majority of the patients..., who demonstrated robust training-induced adaptation, even in elderly heart failure patients," commented the researchers. This study "demonstrates that high-intensity training...is feasible" in older patients "with chronic heart failure and severely impaired cardiovascular function."

Interestingly, only one patient died during the experimental phase, and he was in the moderate-intensity group. The cause of death was found to be "unrelated to exercise training." (It should be noted that all patients were stable and had not had a heart attack in the last 12 months, and that the training took place in a clinical setting. Any patient thinking about trying this should clear it with their doctor beforehand.)

The second study from Norway, reported in *Circulation* (July 7, 2008), again compared moderate-intensity continuous exercise and high-intensity interval training for increasing aerobic capacity (VO2max) and, in addition, for treating metabolic syndrome, a cluster of disorders representing a major risk of coronary heart disease.

Metabolic syndrome has gotten a lot of attention in recent years. Individuals with this syndrome (high blood pressure, high cholesterol, elevated blood sugar, and abdominal obesity) are three times more likely to die of heart disease than healthy people, the researchers explained.

As in the previous study, aerobic interval training (90% of heart-rate maximum) proved more effective than the same volume of moderate continuous exercise (70% of max). Intervals increased VO2max by 35%, compared to 16% for continuous training. This is significant, because individuals with metabolic syndrome usually have reduced fitness. Intervals also did a better job of removing or reducing the risk factors—probably due at least in part to the greater increase in VO2max.

Notably, the Norwegian researchers gave a clear rationale for interval training: "Most evidence suggests that it is the pumping capacity of the heart that limits VO2max and [intervals] enable patients to complete short work periods at higher intensities, which thereby challenge the pumping ability of the heart more than would be possible [with] lower intensities."

In other words, intervals challenge the heart more than steady state exercise. Overload the heart, a muscle, and it grows stronger.

The study included 32 adults (average age 52) with three or more of the metabolic syndrome traits. The difference was that the experimental period was longer than the previous study, 16 weeks compared to 13 weeks.

While both groups experienced a reduction in blood pressure and lost about the same amount of weight, the interval group showed more improvement in how their bodies handle blood sugar and respond to insulin. In addition, the interval group increased HDL "good" cholesterol by about 25%, while the continuous training group showed no improvement.

The researchers concluded that "high-intensity exercise training programs may yield more favorable results [for patients with metabolic syndrome] than programs with low to moderate intensities."

* * *

It appears that high-intensity intervals really are for almost everyone, but they are still not easy. Intervals are fast, effective—and hard.

We'll close this chapter with a study that takes aim at the "intervals are too darn hard" argument—and hits the bull's eye.

Sub-Max Intervals

McMaster University researchers Hood, Little, Tarnopolsky, Myslik, and Gibala have come up with an interval protocol that's suitable for just about anyone, including sedentary individuals. And it works.

Recognizing that going all-out on every interval may be onerous, the McMaster team devised and tested sub-max intervals, a more measured and practical interval protocol. Sub-max intervals are simple in practice, yet sophisticated in effect.

Sub-max intervals are done at 60% of maximum, rather than 100 %. It sounds almost too easy, but it sneaks up on you.

Men and women, average age 45, did six training sessions spread over two weeks. They had not done any regular exercise for at least a year. Each person did 10 one-minute bouts of cycling at about 60% of measured maximum capacity, with one minute recovery between intervals. Resistance remained the same for each interval. Pedal resistance was easy between intervals. Training sessions lasted 20 minutes, plus 3-min warm-up and 5-min cool-down. Blood and muscle samples were taken before training began and 72 hours after the final training session.

Think about it. Every rep was exactly the same and only 60% of capacity. But that's 60% of maximum when rested. The reps become progressively more difficult from rep to rep. You'd expect the heart to beat faster, as fatigue mounted, from rep to rep, and that's what happens. It's what makes the program work.

All subjects completed all prescribed exercise bouts. That's a good sign, because this routine is not exactly a walk in the park. The intervals weren't all out, but they weren't altogether easy either. The effort became demanding at the end—about 95% of heart rate reserve after the last interval. The main difference between this and earlier protocols is that the intervals only become difficult at the end. (A 10-rep set of barbell curls works the same way.)

In spite of the best efforts of the researchers, there's still no free lunch. Effort (overload) was still a necessary part of the plan, but the results were well worth it. The bang for the buck was outstanding!

The major novel finding, according to the researchers, was that six sessions over two weeks improved insulin sensitivity by about 35% and increased muscle mitochondria [oxygen-processing parts of the cell] content by about 35%. Muscle glucose transport capacity increased by about 260%. These markers were selected because they are typically found to be depressed in sedentary individuals.

All of those benefits, from two weeks of training, totaling two hours (plus warm up and cool down), and only a few minutes of it taxing. Wow! That's an amazing demonstration of the power of practical, sub-max interval training.

The results: "A time-efficient strategy to promote mitochondrial biogenesis [a marker of fitness and youthfulness] and induce metabolic adaptations that may reduce the risk for insulin resistance and type 2 diabetes...," the report concluded.

Again, sub-max intervals are hard only at the end. It's easier to go hard with the finish line in sight. Paced properly, it's an invigorating combination of physiology and psychology.

It works. You'll like it. Give it a try.

(The full text of this study was published online in the March, 2011, issue of *Medicine & Science in Sports and Exercise*.)

My experience: I've done sub-max intervals on the Life-cycle, the Airdyne, the Concept 2 Rower, and the Concept 2 Ski Erg—and I really like them. The idea of starting at sub-max intensity and building to maximum intensity on the last rep will work on any interval protocol, including the Tabata 20-10 protocol. It turns "all out" regimens into something people can tolerate—even enjoy.

If you decide to try sub-maximal intervals, you'll wonder how to determine the appropriate speed or load. To do that accurately you'd have to go to an exercise physiology lab at a nearby university or medical facility. That would be time consuming and expensive. I suggest that you experiment a little and then guess. (That's what I have done.)

Give it a trial run on any piece of equipment with a good performance monitor to help you maintain a constant pace or load. Be conservative to start, guess low. If you max-out—or come close—on the last interval you're on the mark. Add speed or load gradually as your fitness improves. Take your time. Don't

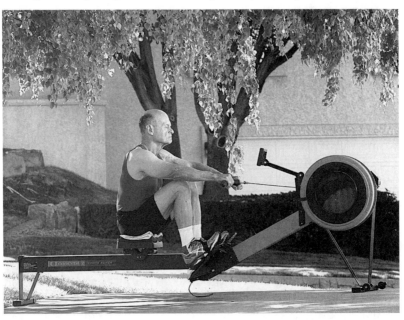

The computerized monitor on the Concept 2 Rower is superb; it shows pace on every stroke and interval. It also counts and recalls pace on each interval, allowing you to track progress from workout to workout. You'll be hard put to find a better vehicle for sub-max intervals.

Photo by Laszlo Bencze

be in a hurry to move up. If you get ahead of yourself, back off and try again. Make it challenging, but not so hard that you flame out before the allotted number of reps. (I've done that. It's no big deal. I simply try again the next workout at a slower pace.)

I suggest doing intervals twice a week—three at most—as part of a balanced training plan. I alternate hard (all-out at the end) and easy (75-80% at the end) intervals, using a variety of equipment (bike, rower, ski erg, treadmill). Hard all the time gets old fast. You'll make better progress with some ebb and flow in your training.

*   *   *

It doesn't get much more exciting than the rise of interval training. But attempting to build aerobic fitness with resistance training is akin to exploring the dark side of the moon. Aerobic-training purists and strength-training skeptics may find it hard to believe, but the science in this area is coming on strong.

We'll look at five breakthrough studies in the next chapter dealing with strength training and aerobic capacity. The first three build basic knowledge. And the last two put the findings into action. That's how the scientific process works. Individual studies add pieces to the puzzle and eventually the whole picture comes into focus.

The outcome is truly exciting, especially for those of us who have been around long enough to see strength training move from basements into the mainstream of fitness. So exciting that, along with Dr. Ralph Carpinelli's breakthrough review, it provided the original stimulus that led me to write this book.

Chapter Four
The Aerobic-Strength Alliance

Strength Training Builds Endurance!

The first study, the Goreham study, bravely challenged the perceived wall between aerobic exercise and strength training. It was brought to my attention by Stuart M. Phillips, PhD, a professor of kinesiology at McMaster University, home to the same people doing the cutting edge research on intervals. The McMaster researchers are also doing ground breaking work on the overlap between the two forms of exercise. (I'll tell you about it in this chapter.)

I asked Professor Phillips about the research in this area. He began by telling me about this 1999 study: "[Goreham and colleagues] showed quite convincingly that resistance trained individuals...showed a number of metabolic changes...that are considered to be a 'hallmark' of aerobic training."

I wanted to learn more—and spread the word.

Traditional wisdom is that aerobic exercise increases oxygen-processing muscle components called mitochondria, and that resistance training builds the contractile fibers (myofibrils). As noted in Chapter 1, the thinking is that muscle gains from resistance training make you stronger, but have little or no effect on endurance; worse, weight-trained muscle is believed to hamper endurance athletes.

Goreham and other researchers from the Kinesiology Department at the University of Waterloo (Ontario, Canada) challenged the orthodoxy. They postulated that muscle mass resulting from heavy resistance training brings with it metabolic changes characteristic of aerobic training. (Heresy!)

To test that theory, they had volunteers do strength training, and then tested their endurance characteristics on stationary bicycles. Specifically, they had untrained males do heavy squats, leg presses, and leg extensions (three sets of 6-8) 3 days a week for 12 weeks. At 4, 7, and 12 weeks they examined metabolic changes using a two-stage, continuous cycling test performed at 57% and 72% of pretraining peak aerobic power (VO2max). Absolute power output and duration (about 56 minutes) was kept the same; nothing was changed from test to test. The goal was to measure metabolic adaptations, if any, resulting from the resistance training. In other words, they sought to determine whether the resistance-trained volunteers became more fit and better able to perform the fixed endurance test.

Importantly, the metabolic changes measured were those generally associated with endurance training. "Regular performance of prolonged [aerobic] exercise results in a well defined series of adaptations in muscle metabolism and substrate utilization," the researchers wrote in introducing the study. "After training, a given submaximal exercise protocol can be performed with less of a *decrease* in high-energy phosphate potential, less of an *increase* in glycogenolysis and glycolysis, and an *increase* in fat utilization." (Emphasis mine)

That's a bit technical, I know, but you get the idea. With prolonged aerobic training, metabolic adaptations occur which make the endurance test easier. The researchers examined those adaptations.

Capillarization (small blood vessel formation) and mitochondrial potential also increase as a result of aerobic training. Traditional thinking is that muscle tissue built with resistance training comes with little or no increase in capillaries and mitochondria. That's at the heart of the belief that resistance-trained muscle hampers endurance. Strength training muscle is looked on as unhelpful baggage.

Goreham found that heavy resistance training (HRT) did, in fact, result in metabolic adaptations usually observed during aerobic exercise. The basic hypothesis was, however, rejected, because the aerobic changes and hypertrophy didn't come together; they came serially, one after the other. As indicated above, the results were nevertheless groundbreaking—and a harbinger of findings to come.

Here's what they found.

1) The metabolic changes were observed only at the higher exercise intensity (72% VO2peak), within the first 4 weeks of training, "and before any changes in fiber cross-sectional area [hypertrophy], capillarization, or oxidative potential."

2) "Additional training for a further 8 weeks failed to exaggerate the metabolic effects that were observed," the researchers continued. "[Nevertheless], the effects of HRT on muscle exercise metabolism, at least qualitatively, are consistent with that which has been reported for prolonged exercise training."

3) There was no change in VO2max.

More surprises were coming, however.

At the 12-week mark Goreham and his colleagues observed an increase in the formation of capillaries sufficient to offset muscle growth. There was no change in capillaries per unit of muscle mass—a good thing.

That was not supposed to happen, of course. As noted earlier, it was thought that muscle tissue built with resistance training comes with little or no increase in capillaries.

One more irregularity remained to be explained. It suggests an important strength component in some forms of endurance, which could be of considerable benefit to many athletes.

Changes that occurred only during the higher-intensity cycling (72% of peak) may have been due in part to training specificity. Dramatic improvements seen in all three strength exercises resurfaced in the high-intensity cycle test results.

In other words, there appeared to be a direct transfer of mechanical strength from resistance training to the higher intensity cycling. Again, this suggests an important strength component in some forms of endurance—in addition to the metabolic adaptations.

A bridge between aerobic and resistant exercise was starting to take shape. Rather than being polar opposites, it was beginning to look like the two forms of exercise are actually complementary.

(The Goreham study was published in March of 1999 in the *American Journal of Physiological Endocrinology and Metabolism*.)

* * *

The McMaster University research mentioned at the beginning of this chapter continued to define the relationship between resistance and aerobic training. By building on the Goreham study, Professor Phillips and his colleagues helped light the way for health professionals, coaches, athletes, and fitness-minded individuals looking for more effective and efficient ways to exercise.

Muscle Carries Aerobic Punch

As we saw in the first chapter and earlier in this chapter, it has been believed that strength training builds muscle at the expense of aerobic conditioning. That it makes people bigger and stronger but doesn't help them resist fatigue. While beneficial to bodybuilders and strength athletes, and providing a cosmetic effect for fitness trainers, it has been said that it has no value to others and, in fact, may be harmful to those with health problems, reducing their stamina. Specifically, exercise physiologists worried that resistance-trained muscles are lacking in mitochondria, the oxygen-processing powerhouses in skeletal muscle.

Researchers at McMaster University are finding that these concerns do not hold up to careful scrutiny.

In 2006, Jason E. Tang, Joseph W. Hartman, and Stuart M. Phillips (Department of Kinesiology, Exercise Metabolism Research Group) investigated "whether or not resistance training induced hypertrophy would reduce the oxidative potential of skeletal muscle." They focused primarily on mitochondrial function in resistance trained muscle mass.

In other words, they were looking into whether muscle growth from strength training limits endurance in athletes and others. It doesn't. Strength training actually appeared to improve aerobic capacity.

"To our knowledge this is the first study to report an increase in oxidative potential and significant hypertrophy [the missing link in the Goreham study] following resistance training," Professor Phillips and his colleagues wrote in the Tang study.

The details of their findings are, of necessity, technical, but the tenor and the results are clear as a bell.

Twelve young men participated in a 12-week resistance training program (whole body, 2-3 sets of 6-12 reps) designed to increase strength and build muscle. The researchers measured the effect of the training program on enzymatic markers of oxygen uptake capacity, and glycolysis (PFK), which plays a role in both aerobic and anaerobic metabolism (with and without oxygen).

Tang and his colleagues expected that the muscle mass created by the resistance training program would maintain its oxygen uptake potential. They were in for a surprise. Resistance training did more; it actually improved aerobic capacity!

"Our results indicate...that muscle [growth] after 12 weeks of high-intensity, whole body, resistance training does not compromise muscle oxidative metabolic potential. Instead, as muscle fiber size increases so too does oxidative enzyme content..., such that muscle oxidative potential is improved after resistance training," Tang et al reported.

Specifically, strength increased an average of 46.5% for all exercises, fat-free muscle mass increased an average of 7.28 pounds, enzymatic markers of oxygen uptake capacity all increased significantly, while glycolysis (PFK) was not affected by training.

"Since the activity of these enzymes are expressed relative to total muscle protein content, these data suggest that the oxidative potential of skeletal muscle is *improved* following resistance training-induced muscle fiber hypertrophy," Tang et al wrote. (Emphasis mine)

"We conclude that resistance training provides a stimulus for improving muscle oxidative potential," Tang and colleagues reported in the journal *Applied Physiology Nutrition and Metabolism*, Vol. 31, 2006.

Moreover—this is a significant insight—the McMaster researchers observed that their conclusion had been heralded by their finding the previous year that sprint intervals build endurance. As we saw in the last chapter, they found that bouts of very hard 30 second sprints can stimulate marked improvements in aerobic capacity after as little as 2 weeks of training.

"Taken together," they wrote, "these findings illustrate how short-duration high-intensity exercise can stimulate adaptations in oxidative metabolism that have traditionally been associated with only endurance exercise."

The estrangement between aerobic training and resistance training was beginning to thaw. The bridge between aerobic and strength training was getting stronger, adding structural integrity.

"I think it's fair to say that there is a lot more in common between aerobic training and resistance training than we've been taught," Jason Tang's colleague and senior researcher Stuart Phillips wrote in a personal communication.

The Goreham and Tang studies—along with the new findings on interval training—taken together, make a powerful case for short, hard training as a key element in a program for total fitness. Scientists were beginning to understand that brief high-intensity training—intervals and strength training—provides advantages once thought impossible.

Were endurance athletes and fitness trainers listening? I don't know, but I sure am.

Hang with me. There's a lot more to learn.

Strength Training Builds Muscle— and Mitochondria

To recap, the Goreham study in 1999 found that heavy strength training stimulated metabolic changes that are considered to be a 'hallmark' of aerobic training. Seven years later, Tang reported an increase in aerobic potential *and* significant hypertrophy following strength training. (Hypertrophy was the missing element in the Goreham study.)

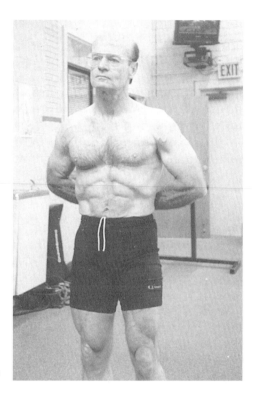

Carl Miller, United States weightlifting coach at the Montreal Olympic Games, has long believed that strength training builds total fitness. He has had great success teaching athletic-type lifting for total fitness to all ages at his fitness center in Santa Fe, New Mexico, where this photo was taken after a workout.

Photo by Carl Miller

Two years later, in 2008, Wilkinson and colleagues broke new ground with a finding that strength training increased the formation of mitochondria, the kingpins of aerobic fitness. Earlier studies had found *markers* of mitochondrial growth.

Importantly, the ability to use oxygen to convert nutrients to energy depends on the number, size, and efficiency of the mitochondria in the muscle. If strength training increases mitochondria this is big news for athletes and fitness trainers looking for a competitive edge.

To test their hypothesis that a single bout of strength training would stimulate growth of both strength and endurance fibers, Wilkinson devised a unique protocol. It would not be practical in a gym setting, but was ideal for the experiment, and really quite novel.

Ten untrained men (average age 20.5 years) did knee extensions with one leg and cycling with the other leg; the two forms of exercise were done on separate days. The men were tested at rest before the exercise began, after a single bout of each exercise, and at the end of the 10 week program.

The participants were their own controls, because one limb

was assigned to strength exercise and the other limb to endurance exercise. Comparing metabolic responses in the same person gave the study increased statistical power.

Clearly, Wilkinson and her colleagues wanted to understand the interplay between the two forms of exercise. To do that, they measured the rate of myofibrillar and mitochondrial protein formation in both limbs.

"We observed that in untrained muscle, resistance exercise stimulated both myofibrillar and muscle mitochondrial protein synthesis [formation]," Wilkinson's team reported. "*We contend that this is the first study to report an increase of human muscle mitochondrial protein synthesis after acute* [short, hard] *exercise.*" (Emphasis mine)

"Resistance exercise stimulated both myofibrillar and mitochondrial protein synthesis, 67% and 69%, respectively," they reported. In short, strength and endurance elements responded equally to the first bout of strength training—as predicted.

After 10 weeks, strength training (knee extensions) stimulated an additional 36% increase in the formation of the contractile fibers; the muscles were getting bigger and stronger. Endurance training (cycling), on the other hand, stimulated a 154% increase of mitochondrial protein formation after the first workout, and 105% after 10 weeks of training. Endurance training, however, stimulated only the endurance component. It did not stimulate growth in the contractile fibers—at any time.

The new finding is that strength training initially stimulated growth in *both* the strength and the endurance elements in the thigh, while endurance training stimulated growth in only the endurance elements, in trained and untrained muscle. Endurance training is more specific—and limited—than resistance training.

(For more details—and there are many—consult the full report: Wilkinson et al, *Journal of Physiology* 586.15 (2008) pp 3701-3717)

* * *

Professor Stuart M. Phillips, who was also involved in the last study, commented meaningfully in a personal communication on the findings in the three studies we've been discussing.

"The perceived divergence and 'exclusivity' of response with each form of training – i.e., aerobic training begets mitochondria and resistance training leads to muscle hypertrophy – is, we think, incorrect. The responses lie instead along a continuum and yet you cannot have one without some of the other. It

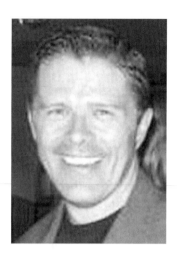

Stuart M. Phillips, PhD, a professor of kinesiology at McMaster University, is a leader in studying the synergy between resistance and aerobic training.
Photo courtesy of Phillips

is true enough that when practiced for long periods of time that the phenotype becomes more specialized, but is this due 100% to training or that the training allowed you to express some underlying genetic potential for adaptation? Some people are just born runners and others lifters in my view!"

* * *

"Some people are just born runners and others lifters in my view!" So true. Phil Heath, the 2011 and 2012 Mr. Olympia, would be wasting his time trying to win the Boston Marathon. By the same token, Kenya's Geoffrey Mutai, who won the 2011 Boston Marathon in record time, would be out of place on stage at the Olympia; he would be equally hopeless in the "World's Strongest Man" competition.

In truth, most of us would be out of place in either venue.

While my phenotype is less clear, I've known since my teen years that I prefer lifting to running. I was a good wrestler in high school—due mainly to lifting—but I hated the mandatory run around the football field after practice. My dad was the same way; he was good at pole vaulting, jumping, and throwing the discus, but had no interest (or aptitude) in running distance.

Most people are probably in the middle or tilt a little one way or the other. After you exercise for a while, you'll have a pretty good idea where you fall on the spectrum between strength and endurance. We almost always enjoy what we do best. Few people are willing to do things they don't enjoy for very long.

Dr. Kenneth Cooper's book *Aerobics*, discussed in Chapter 1, convinced me that aerobic exercise is important. Carol and I

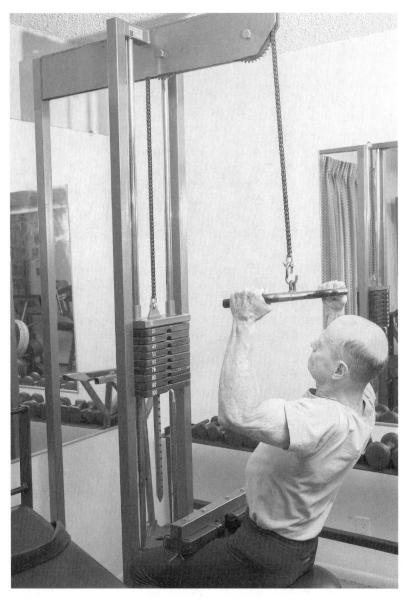

I've known since my teen years that I prefer lifting to running.

Photo by Laszlo Bencze

have been doing some form of aerobic exercise ever since, some running, but mostly biking, hiking, and walking. Still, I was never really into aerobic exercise—until I discovered indoor rowing and later interval training. Rowing and interval training excited me, because they offered the option of doing short, hard workouts, akin to lifting. They have a major strength component. That's what I enjoy and do best; it's my thing.

I have plenty of company. Many people just can't get excited about jogging and the like, probably because there's no challenge or they're not very good at it. They end up doing aerobic exercise sporadically or not at all. Many never find a form of aerobic exercise that they enjoy and do well. The same goes for strength training; some people find it unappealing. Fortunately, new options are opening up in both forms of exercise.

For example, men and women who can't see themselves lifting heavy weights are discovering effort based lifting, which provides the same benefits with light weights or other forms of resistance training. (See Chapter 2)

We need both strength and endurance to be totally fit and healthy, and we can almost always achieve both in ways that suit our body and personality—through regular training or other methods when we are pressed for time.

The new findings on the synergy between resistance and endurance exercise open up training options that make it easier to become totally fit and healthy.

Knowledge is power—find the way or ways that suit you best.

* * *

You can see why I'm excited about these studies; they are expanding our understanding of the benefits of strength training

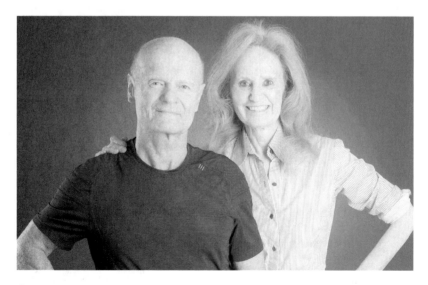

Carol and I have been doing some form of aerobic exercise for over 40 years. *Photo by Pat Berrett*

in ways once considered unthinkable. More scientists, it seems, are plumbing the intricate workings of the human body under stress. As a trainer and student for over 50 years, I'm energized. We are learning things about training apace; things that are expanding our options like never before.

Primed to learn more, let's move on to the last two studies, one from Sweden and the other from McMaster University in Canada. Scientists are looking for ways to take advantage of the synergy between resistance and aerobic training. Both studies examined the effect of combining the two forms of exercise. We'll start with the Swedish breakthrough.

Combination Training Works

Li Wang and colleagues predicted that the effect of endurance training would be impaired by the addition of strength training. They were in for a nice surprise.

The study design was straightforward, something you could envision endurance athletes actually doing.

Ten healthy subjects performed either endurance exercise (1 hour of cycling at 65% of peak capacity) or endurance exercise followed by resistance exercise (1 hour cycling + 6 sets of leg presses with 70 to 80% of 1 repetition maximum). The first group was labelled E, and the second group E+R.

Muscle biopsies obtained before and after exercise for both groups (E and E+R) were tested for specific markers, which told the researchers precisely what was happening inside the muscles. Earlier studies had relied on performance—changes in endurance or strength—which would provide only limited information on the underlying adaptations and mechanisms involved.

Laboratory experiments involving skeletal muscle in rats had shown that interference in molecular signalling may occur if both types of exercise are employed. Human reaction, however, has been undefined. Would strength training disrupt adaptation to endurance training in humans? "It is unclear," Wang et al wrote.

"The aim of the present study was to investigate if resistance exercise can alter the molecular signalling response to endurance exercise in skeletal muscle," the Wang team wrote. "We hypothesized that the addition of resistance exercise would reduce the response to endurance exercise in the expression of marker genes related to mitochondrial biogenesis."

They were mistaken! The molecular markers increased with

both E and E+R, "*but the mRNA levels were about twofold higher after E+R,*" Wang et al reported. (Emphasis mine)

"Contrary to our hypothesis, the results demonstrate that [resistance exercise] performed after endurance exercise amplifies the adaptive signalling response of mitochondrial biogenesis... The results suggest that concurrent training may be beneficial for the adaptation of muscle oxidative capacity," they concluded.

Here's their take–away message for athletes and fitness trainers.

"The results from this study challenge the current view of how to optimize endurance training and indicate that a bout of resistance exercise performed shortly after endurance exercise can improve the training-induced stimulation of mitochondrial biogenesis," the researchers added in discussing their findings. They also speculated that high-intensity sprints, intervals, might produce a "similar boost effect."

"Another interesting finding," Wang et al added, "was that endurance exercise had only a small influence on the signalling pathway promoting protein synthesis." In other words, the hour of cycling didn't interfere with the response to the leg presses. It was a win-win combination.

Again, we see the limited—and specific—effect of steady state endurance training, along with the synergistic effect of strength training.

The Wang study was published in the November, 2011, *Journal of Applied Physiology*.

* * *

Taking it a step further, the Wang study suggests to me that a short series of intervals at the end of a strength training workout (something I employ regularly) may boost strength *and* endurance. Keep in mind that hard intervals (unlike steady state aerobics) activate fast twitch fibers while building endurance.

The second study, from McMaster University, tests a variation of that idea by comparing strength and endurance training separately, and back to back on the same day. Professor Stuart Phillips was once again deeply involved.

More Bang for the Buck

The McMaster University researchers and colleagues in Australia, New Zealand, and the UK had sedentary volunteers perform three separate trails on different days. On one day, the men rode a stationary cycle for 40 minutes at a moderate pace.

On another day, they did eight hard sets of knee extensions. In the third and final session, they did four sets of knee extensions followed by 20 minutes on the stationary cycle. (Note that volume was cut in half for both forms of exercise on the combination training day.)

Biopsies were obtained before and after each trial.

Again, doing both weights and aerobics on the same day produced a surprise. It turned out to have a delightful advantage.

"The current study data indicates that concurrent training is as effective as either isolated mode in stimulating acute myofibrillar and mitochondrial protein synthesis rates," the researchers wrote. "Importantly, the increases...occurred despite the completion of only 50% of the workload performed in each of the isolated resistance exercise and aerobic exercise modes," they added.

Stuart Phillips, who oversaw the study, said his team expected that "we would see a greater response to each exercise individually," but that didn't happen. Instead, after combined training, the men's muscles displayed the same amount of change within both cellular pathways as after either type of exercise on its own—even though the men had actually completed only half as much of each. "We saw no indication of interference," he told *New York Times* fitness writer Gretchen Reynolds.

"It appears that you can set up a workout regimen that happens to be convenient for you...and you're not going to get less training response," Phillips said. Best of all, he explained, the men did only half as much cycling and lifting. "But their muscles couldn't tell the difference."

Combine weights and aerobics on the same day if that suits your schedule and energy level; the results may surprise you.

The Canadian study, co-authored by Cheyne E. Donges and Nicholas A. Burd, was published April 5, 2012, in *The Journal of Applied Physiology*.

* * *

Take away message for this chapter: The estrangement between strength and endurance training has long been a part of exercise lore; my high school coach told me that real athletes don't lift weights. Few coaches would say that today, but the tension remains. This chapter challenges the traditional view that strength and endurance training don't mix. The studies presented here strongly suggest that the two forms of training are, in fact, complementary.

Professor Stuart Phillips (who was involved in the Tang,

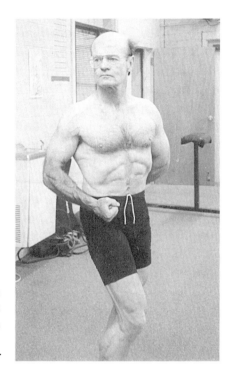

My high school coach told me not to lift weights. I wish he could see the results these many years later.

Photo by Carl Miller

Wilkinson, and Donges-Burd studies) is convinced. He wrote in a recent e-mail, "I am quite certain for all but the most ardent powerlifters (i.e., 1-2 reps/sets) that multiple sets of resistance exercise promote mitochondrial expansion!"

If you want strength and endurance, multiple sets of resistance training is one way—new to most—to achieve that goal. Brief, hard, and infrequent resistance training combined with interval training is another way. Steady state endurance training combined with conventional resistance training is still another way.

Taking charge means doing what works best for you.

* * *

Now let's turn to the body's pilot—the brain.

The Greeks were right about the ideal of a sound mind in a sound body. The stereotype of a strong back and a weak mind is way off the mark. I've long believed that a strong mind and a strong body go hand in hand. But it wasn't until the last decade or so that I began studying the new science of exercise and the brain. The evidence is strong, and growing stronger, that both resistance and aerobic exercise improve mental function. The research is coming at a remarkable pace. In the next chapter we'll talk about some of the most exciting discoveries.

Chapter Five

Exercise and The Brain

Train Your Brain

My first exposure to the science of exercise and the brain was as a participant in the University of New Mexico Aging Study. Professor Mark A. McDaniel, chairman of the UNM Psychology Department, spoke at the annual meeting of the Aging Study. He was collaborating on a book on aging and memory with Professor Giles O. Einstein, chairman of the psychology department at Furman University, and asked for topic suggestions from the audience. I said I'd like to know more about the effects of physical exercise. I didn't think anything more about it until I received a letter from McDaniel and Einstein announcing that their book was completed and available in bookstores.

Their book, *Memory Fitness: A Guide to Successful Aging* (Yale University Press, 2004), was my introduction to the notion of training the brain. I was thrilled to read that, in the authors' opinion, when it comes to maximizing both your physical and mental functioning, "It is downright risky behavior not to exercise."

A few concepts are basic and well accepted.

"There is complete agreement today that when training is built up gradually and done properly, it is dangerous not to exercise," one of the authors wrote. That was not always his view, however. Influenced by the death of a favorite teacher while shoveling snow, he subscribed to the traditional view that people over 50 should take it easy and conserve their fleeting resources. His research for the book turned him into "an impassioned crusader for the value of exercise in older adulthood."

The first and most obvious benefit of exercise is emotional well-being. We tend to be depressed more often as we age. According to the authors, about 15% of older adults report feeling depressed. Unfortunately, the suicide rate goes up with age.

One factor that contributes to depression, according to McDaniel and Einstein, is a sense of losing control of our lives. We can't do the things we once could, and we're forced to depend on others. Exercise helps to alleviate the problem. "To the extent that exercise enables you to maintain your physical capabilities," the authors explained, "this should positively affect your sense of personal control and thus your emotional outlook on life—with the result that depression may be reduced or avoided altogether."

Other benefits of exercise on the brain are more specific.

Endurance or aerobic exercise increases blood flow and oxy-

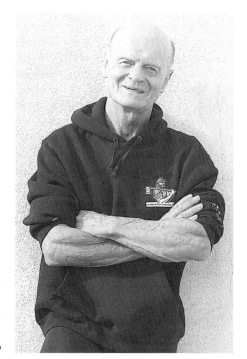

Staying fit with exercise improves your outlook on life.
It makes you happier and
more productive.
Photo by Laszlo Bencze

gen to the brain, resulting in improved cognitive function. "Cardiovascular exercise has been shown to increase the stroke volume of the heart and oxygen transportation to the brain," the
authors wrote. Exercise also appears to stimulate new capillary
growth in the brain, which would allow more oxygen to reach
brain cells.

In one "provocative" study cited by the authors, younger and
older rats were raised in an environment that encouraged exercise, but not intellectual stimulation. Another group was given
intellectual stimulation but not allowed to exercise. Interestingly, the rats that exercised showed more capillary development
in the brain, but those given intellectual stimulation showed
more neuronal development (synaptic connections, receptor
sites, etc.). "These data strongly suggest that exercise imparts
important advantages to the brains of both younger and older
animals," Einstein and McDaniel related. Exercise and intellectual stimulation appear to work together to improve brain
function.

We know that exercise improves oxygen flow to the brain, but
does it actually benefit cognitive functioning? Researchers have
addressed this issue from more than one angle. First, they compared cognitive function of people who exercise regularly with

sedentary people of the same age. "The majority of studies show that exercisers perform better on cognitive tasks than non-exercisers," reported the authors. "Most exciting, the pattern of results suggests that exercise may confer the most benefit on the kinds of mental tasks that are most affected by aging." For example, aging tends to reduce the ability to retrieve information from memory without using cues (essay questions versus multiple choice). "Exercise may protect against this reduction," said the authors.

Still, the difference in memory could be due to something other than exercise. Maybe people who exercise take better care of themselves or perhaps they are genetically less affected by aging. To answer this question scientists use the experimental approach. They take groups of sedentary older people and put half of them on an exercise program for several months, and then compare the groups on various cognitive tests. "Experiments of this sort have shown that exercise can produce substantial benefits on some tasks but not others," reported the authors.

An examination of prior studies found that exercise mainly helped individuals perform tasks controlled by the frontal lobes of the brain. "This is interesting," the authors wrote, "because there is strong evidence today that our frontal lobes show the earliest and greatest amount of age associated losses." According to the authors, the frontal lobes are thought to be responsible for working memory (keeping information in mind while being distracted) and executive control processes (planning and coordinating complex tasks).

Studies specifically designed to confirm this hypothesis, according to Einstein and McDaniel, show that groups performing aerobic exercise do in fact demonstrate significant improvements in tasks thought to involve the frontal lobes, but not in other tasks. Significantly, the mental abilities most improved by aerobic exercise are those that appear to be most negatively affected by aging.

Research on exercise and mental functioning is "increasing at a feverish pace," the authors reported. Most of the research to date has involved aerobic exercise, but the effect of strength training is now being explored. Encouragingly, it was reported in 2001 "that the benefits of exercise on memory are greater when people mix resistance training with cardiovascular training and with intense cardiovascular exercise relative to moderate exercise."

Hmmm, sounds familiar.

*   *   *

The next important event in my education on this topic was the publication of Dr. John J. Ratey's life changing book *SPARK: The Revolutionary New Science of Exercise and the Brain* (Little, Brown, 2008). Ratey, a clinical professor of psychiatry at the Harvard School of Medicine, didn't mince words. "Exercise is the single most powerful tool you have to optimize your brain function," he trumpeted.

Reboot Your Brain with Exercise

Ratey begins the book by telling how a revolutionary PE program helped make the 19,000 kids in a suburban school district outside of Chicago perhaps the fittest in the nation—and first in the world in science. This remarkable and uplifting case study is one of the *sparks* that inspired him to write the book.

The core idea of the program is exemplified by "Zero Hour PE," a new physical education class scheduled before first period. "The object of Zero Hour was to determine whether working out before school gives these kids a boost in reading ability and in the rest of their subjects," Ratey explained.

There are many other aspects of the overall program, of course, but the main thing to understand is that this is not the typical team-oriented curriculum. The emphasis is on fitness instead of sports. The kids are encouraged to find an activity they enjoy. Eighteen choices are offered, ranging from rock climbing to aerobic dance. The idea is to find something that allows a student to experience success.

It worked. The kids got fitter *and* smarter.

The kids in Zero Hour were sent off to their first period class in a "state of heightened awareness" and prepared to learn. At the end of the semester, they showed a 17 percent improvement in reading and comprehension, compared with a 10.7 percent improvement for students who opted to sleep in and take the standard PE class.

The "New PE" curriculum produced eye popping results district wide. On a test designed to compare students' knowledge levels from different countries in math and science, district students finished sixth in math—and, as noted earlier, number one in the world in science. Now, that's success!

Two of the coaches gave the shorthand explanation: "In our department, we create the brain cells. It's up to the other teachers to fill them." Obviously, both did their job extremely well.

As suggested in the last section, exercise alone won't make you smarter; it preps your mind to learn. You also have to study.

The case gets better, more concrete and convincing, as Ratey continued to present and explain the evidence for the physical exercise-brain connection.

"In addition to priming our state of mind," Ratey related, "exercise influences learning directly, at the cellular level, improving the brain's potential to log on and process new information."

It is now clear that the brain is flexible or malleable; neuroscientists call it plastic. Everything we do, think, or feel shapes our brain. "[The brain] is an adaptable organ that can be molded by input in much the same way as a muscle can be sculpted by lifting a barbell," Ratey told readers. "The more you use it, the stronger it becomes."

Over the past 15 or so years, Ratey related, a family of proteins loosely called *factors* have "dramatically changed our understanding of connections in the brain, specifically how they develop and grow." The most prominent is brain-derived neurotrophic factor (BDNF). "Whereas neurotransmitters carry out signaling," Ratey explained, "neurotrophins such as BDNF build and maintain the cell circuitry—the infrastructure itself."

A massive amount of research, said Ratey, has shown that BDNF "nourishes neurons [brain cells] like fertilizer." When researchers sprinkle BDNF onto neurons in the lab, the cells spontaneously sprout new branches, producing the same structural growth required for learning—causing Ratey to think of BDNF as "Miracle-Gro for the brain."

That's exciting, but what really *sparked* Ratey's interest was the discovery that, in mice, exercise elevates Miracle-Gro throughout the brain. For years, he had been a vocal proponent of using exercise for many psychological issues, based on what he had seen in his patients. "But this was different," he wrote. "By showing that exercise sparks the master molecule of the learning process, [researchers] nailed down a direct biological connection between movement and cognitive function. In so doing, [they] blazed the trail for the study of exercise in neuroscience."

That finding laid the foundation for proving that exercise strengthens the cellular machinery of learning. "BDNF gives the synapses the tools they need to take in information, process it, remember it, and put it in context," Ratey wrote.

Exercise alone, however, won't make anyone a genius. As one

neuroscientist put it, "With learning, you have to respond to something in a different way. But something has to be there." Exercise creates an environment conducive to learning, but you must give your brain a new challenge.

"If we don't use the newborn neurons," says Ratey, "we lose them."

So, it's up to you to do the exercise *and* challenge your brain. Okay, you say, how do I go about doing that? What's the best exercise program?

Your options are many; they include most of the things we've been talking about in earlier chapters. I'll give you an overview of what Ratey suggested in the book. Dr. Ratey's guidelines are flexible. He told me in a personal communication that he welcomes suggestions.

"The best advice," Ratey advised, "is to get fit and then continue challenging [yourself]. If you get your body in shape, your mind will follow....We know with certainty that having a normal body mass index and a robust cardiovascular system optimizes your brain."

That's the bottom line; there's no magic exercise formula for brain fitness; there are many that will do the job quite well.

Dr. Ratey recommends some form of exercise six days a week, mostly aerobic exercise, but strength training as well. At least two days should be intense; to allow recovery, these days should not be back to back.

Moderate days can be walking. This will increase blood flow, and, with that, Ratey wrote, "comes the chemical cascade that produces serotonin, brain-derived neurotrophic factor (BDNF), and other nourishing molecules." Work up to an hour, increasing the pace as your fitness improves. Don't overdo, however; because the moderate aerobic days help you recover from the hard days.

Hard days, Ratey warned, should only be added after you have developed a base of fitness. Consult your doctor, if you have concerns about your readiness. When you are ready, the benefits are surprising—even to Dr. Ratey.

If you want to really challenge yourself, you can mix in short interval sprints. "One of the key differences between moderate and high-intensity exercise," Ratey wrote, "is that once you get closer to your maximum, and especially when you get into the anaerobic range, the pituitary gland in your brain unleashes human growth hormone (HGH)."

"HGH is the body's master craftsman," he explained, "burning belly fat, layering on muscle fiber, and pumping up brain volume. Researchers believe it can reverse the loss of brain volume that naturally occurs as you age."

He continued: "Normally HGH stays in the bloodstream only a few minutes, but a session of sprinting can keep the level elevated for up to four hours. In the brain, HGH balances neurotransmitter levels and boosts the production of all the growth factors I've mentioned....It gets into the very cell nucleus and switches on genes that crank up the mechanisms of neuronal growth."

Interval training was new to Ratey. "Two days a week," he related, "I started including a handful of sprints during my treadmill runs, and let me tell you, they hurt. Just writing about it makes me cringe a little, but it was well worth the effort. After one month of this business, I lost the final ten pounds I'd been after for years—it peeled right off my midsection."

Twice a week, he now does just twenty minutes of jogging, interspersed with five sprints of twenty to thirty seconds each in which "I run as fast as I can."

Dr. Ratey also recommended strength training, even though the research was skimpy at the time of his writing. (We'll talk about new research on strength training and brain function below.)

"One factor clearly affected by strength training is HGH," he reported. A recent study found that "doing squats doubled

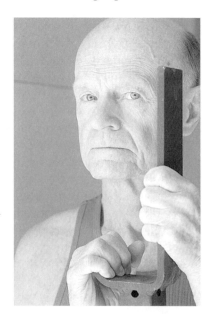

You must continue challenging your body—and your mind.
Photo by Laszlo Bencze

HGH levels compared with running at high intensity for thirty minutes."

"I think this will turn out to have important implications for exercise recommendations," he wrote.

What Ratey himself does is instructive: "Weights plus crunches and balance exercises two times a week." Two other days, he does 40 minutes on the elliptical trainer; and finally, two days of 20 minutes on the treadmill with intervals. He challenges his body—and his brain—in a variety of ways.

Summing up his regimen, he wrote: "I'm doing everything I can to keep my prefrontal cortex, and everything it's connected to, pumped up."

That's what taking charge is about.

* * *

Professors McDaniel, Einstein, and Ratey predicted that strength training would play a larger part of future exercise recommendations—and that is what we are seeing.

Both Aerobics and Weights Boost Brain Power

While most of the research on exercise and cognitive function has involved aerobic exercise, the effects of strength training are now being explored. Experts believe the greatest benefits may occur when aerobic exercise is paired with resistance training.

A community observation study from Germany found that regular physical activity is associated with a lower risk of cognitive impairment. A second study, from Canada, found that once-a-week progressive-resistance training improved cognitive skills in senior women. Both studies were published in the January 25, 2010, issue of the *Archives of Internal Medicine*.

The first study, led by Thorleif Etgen, MD, Department of Psychiatry and Psychotherapy at a university in Munich, Germany, examined data collected on 3903 people (age 55 or older) every 3 months for two years. Participants completed a cognitive impairment test and a questionnaire that divided them by activity level: none (584), moderate (1523), and high (1796).

Moderate activity was defined as vigorous activities (including walking, hiking, biking, and swimming) performed less than 3 days a week. High activity was defined as 3 or more days a week.

At the time of enrollment, 418 participants (10.7%) had cognitive impairment. Of these, 21.4% were in the no activity group, compared to 10.5% and 7.3% in the moderate and high activity groups, respectively.

At the end of two years, the researchers found that 207 additional people (5.9%) had developed impairment. The new impairment group included 13.9% with no physical activity, but only 6.7% and 5.1% with moderate and high activity.

Dr. Etgen was amazed by the magnitude of the findings. "Physical activity cut in half the odds of developing incident cognitive impairment. We were also surprised that moderate physical activity had nearly the same effect as high physical activity."

"The take-home message is: Keep on moving," said Etgen.

Positive results like these for aerobic activity prompted researchers from Vancouver General Hospital and the Department of Physical Therapy at the University of British Columbia to examine the cognitive benefits of resistance training.

In introducing the second study, the researchers noted that an earlier analysis had found that "the greatest benefit of aerobic exercise on cognition occurred when it was paired with resistance training." They sought to explore the "spectrum of cognitive functions" improved as a result of once or twice a week resistance training.

"To our knowledge, no study to date has examined the minimum frequency of resistance training required for cognitive benefits," wrote lead researcher Teresa Liu-Ambrose, PhD, PT, and her colleagues.

Her team enrolled 155 community-dwelling women (age 65 to 75) and randomly assigned them to once-weekly (54) or twice-weekly (52) resistance training classes, or a control group (54) doing twice-weekly balance and toning classes. The classes were for 12 months.

Significantly, the resistance training protocol was high intensity, a departure from the high volume protocol seen in most studies. All major body parts were covered, from the large muscles of the lower body to the smaller muscles of the upper body. Two sets of 6 to 8 reps were performed for each exercise. Resistance was increased when 2 sets of 6 to 8 reps were completed with "proper form and without discomfort." The number of sets completed and the load lifted for each exercise were recorded for each participant at every class.

The balance and toning classes consisted of stretching, range of motion exercises, exercises to strengthen the pelvic floor muscles, balance exercises, and relaxation techniques. Other than bodyweight, no additional loading was applied.

All participants took an executive function test of selective attention and conflict resolution, and a task performance test. Gait speed was also measured.

Both resistance training groups significantly improved their performance on the executive function test compared to the balance and toning group. Task performance improved by 12.6% and 10.9% in the once-weekly and twice-weekly resistance training groups, respectively; the skill deteriorated by 0.5% in the balance and toning control group.

"To our knowledge, this is the first study to demonstrate that engaging in progressive resistance training as infrequently as once a week can significantly benefit executive cognitive function in...senior women," Liu-Ambrose and her colleagues wrote.

Finally, enhanced selective attention and conflict resolution was significantly associated with increased gait speed. "This finding was quite clinically relevant because walking speed is a big indicator of a person's general well-being and also a predictor of mortality," Liu-Ambrose explained.

Liu-Ambrose urged that resistance training be more widely promoted. "Exercise is currently promoted clinically but I think it's typically more, 'Take more walks.' But there's a lot of emerging evidence that shows that resistance training not only has similar benefits as aerobic training, but it also has very specific benefits."

In an editorial comment, Marco Pahor, MD, professor, Department of Aging and Geriatrics, University of Florida, wrote: "Both studies [German and Canadian] provide very promising evidence that physical activity *in any form* can improve cognitive function...Both studies are extremely compelling and set the stage for larger multicenter trials to come."

* * *

A three-pronged approach—diet, aerobics, and weights—is the formula for total fitness. I've been saying that for more than three decades. I believe we can now safely add that "total fitness" includes brain fitness. Professors McDaniel and Einstein were correct that the benefits of exercise on mental function are greater when people mix resistance training with cardiovascular training. Dr. Ratey said essentially the same thing.

Knowledge and action, taking charge, can make us fit in body and mind.

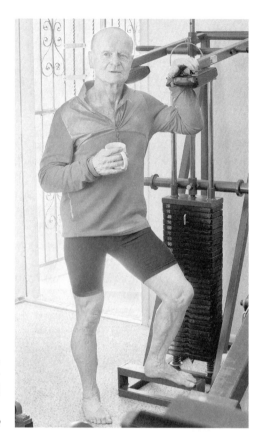

A balanced approach, aerobic exercise and resistance training, is best for body—and mind.
Photo by Laszlo Bencze

* * *

Late breaking news on BDNF shows that the case for exercise is growing stronger and stronger; it's a fitting way to end this chapter. The news is very encouraging for those of us who want to train our brain in the most effective and efficient way; it reinforces the view that brief exercise is effective in preserving and improving mental function.

Miracle-Gro for the Brain

Not long ago, a mention of brain-derived neurotrophic factor (BDNF) would have elicited a blank stare from all but neuroscientists. Dr. John Ratey, as we saw, changed that with the publication of his mass-market book *SPARK* in 2008. He captured the imagination of readers by terming BDNF "Miracle-Gro for the brain." Everyone could see that image in their mind's eye. BDNF nourishes brain cells like fertilizer; it makes them sprout new branches. As Ratey explained, BDNF creates the infrastructure for learning.

What really *sparked* Ratey's interest, however, was a report that, in mice, exercise elevates BDNF throughout the brain. "[That finding] laid the foundation for proving that exercise strengthens the cellular machinery of learning," Ratey wrote. "BDNF gives the synapses the tools they need to take in information, process it, remember it, and put it in context."

A few months ago as this is written, an article by Gretchen Reynolds in *The New York Times* triggered renewed interest in exercise and BDNF. Reynolds reported on four studies, all published in 2011, which zero-in on how exercise stimulates BDNF—and brain function. The new studies involve humans as well as rodents and come from around the world: Ireland, Brazil, and two from the USA.

In the first study (published in the journal *Physiological Behavior*), scientists from the School of Medicine at the University of Dublin gave sedentary male students a series of memory tests, before exercise, and again after exercise. They found a chain reaction: exercise, BDNF, learning, and memory. What's more, the form of exercise that brought about the improvement was a surprise, a first.

Before exercise, all of the students watched a rapidly moving lineup of photos with the faces and names of strangers. After a 30-minute break, they were all asked to match the faces and the names.

The memory test was then repeated after three different stationary bicycle protocols: a single bout of intense exercise, three weeks of moderate-intensity aerobic training, and five weeks of the same regimen. The single bout of exercise had the students pedal against gradually increasing resistance until voluntary exhaustion. The three and five week programs consisted of traditional steady state exercise.

Blood samples were taken throughout the experiment to measure circulating amounts of BDNF. Rested volunteers did not register any change in BDNF—or improvement in memory. Notably, two of the exercise groups showed an increase in both.

"The results show that a short period of high-intensity cycling results in enhancements in performance of the face-name matching," the researcher reported. "These changes in cognitive function were paralleled by increased concentration of BDNF... in the serum of exercising subjects." Surprisingly, three weeks of steady-state cycle training had no effect, but five weeks did.

"Increases in fitness, cognitive function and serum BDNF response...were observed following 5 weeks of aerobic training."

"To our knowledge, this is the first evidence for an acute exercise-induced enhancement in [memory] in humans," the researchers wrote in their report. "It is possible that the effect of chronic exercise on cognition may be mediated by an alternative mechanism involving BDNF," they added. In other words, both long and short exercise improve memory, possibly in different ways.

The second and third studies involved rodents.

The second study was another test of brief exercise. Brazilian scientists ran sedentary elderly rats at an easy pace on a treadmill for four to six minutes several days a week for five weeks—and then compared the exercised rats to much younger rats on rodent memory tests. They then analyzed changes in the heart, skeletal muscle, and brain tissue of the exercised old rats. The findings were nothing short of spectacular.

Not only did this very conservative exercise program increase the oxygen capacity of their muscles and hearts, it reversed age-related learning and memory impairment. "Remarkably, the observed cognitive-enhancing properties of short bouts of exercise were accompanied by [a cascade of reactions in the memory center of their brains] that culminates in the marked increase of... BDNF protein levels," the researchers wrote in summarizing their findings. (The study was published in the journal *Mechanisms of Ageing and Development*.)

The third study focused on BDNF formation in the brains of exercising rodents. The exercise was spontaneous and unprogramed.

While it has been shown repeatedly that exercise improves brain function in conjunction with the action of BDNF, the mechanisms involved have remained unclear. To learn more about the process involved scientists in the Brain Injury Research Center at UCLA studied changes in the brain of rats allowed to run freely for seven days. What they found was illuminating: the memory centers of the free-running rats teemed with developing BDNF and mature BDNF not found in sedentary rats. Among other things, they found what appeared to be an orderly progression in the formation of BDNF following exercise.

The UCLA team concluded: "Exercise appears to act as an excellent homeostatic regulator of BDNF processing and function with important implications for brain plasticity." In other words, exercise keeps the level of BDNF within a range that would be likely to optimize brain function. (This study was published in the journal *Neuroscience*.)

Finally, Reynolds wrote about the role of BDNF in the skill level of aging pilots. Reynolds called it "perhaps the most inspiring of the recent experiments." It brings the spotlight back around to humans in a real life situation.

Researchers at Stanford's School of Medicine studied experienced pilots ages 40 to 69 who took standardized flight simulation tests three or more times over a two year period. Importantly, they examined them for a specific structural change in their brain BDNF to determine if it correlated with flight simulation scores. In addition, they measured hippocampal volume in some of the pilots.

They found that the structural change in BDNF did, in fact, predict the rate of decline in cockpit performance scores. They also found that age-related changes in hippocampal volume were significantly altered by the structure of their BDNF.

All of the pilots declined somewhat in cockpit performance over the two-year period. A similar decline with age is common in all of us. In this case, however, the decline was most striking in a particular group carrying a gene variant known to reduce BDNF in the brain.

Dr. Ahmad Salehi, an associate professor of psychiatry at Stanford and senior author of the study, told Reynolds that his team plans next to examine the exercise histories of the pilots to see if those with the gene variant responded differently to exercise. Salehi believes that exercise would be especially important to those with the variant. "But for everyone," he emphasized, "the evidence is very, very strong that physical activity will increase BDNF levels and improve cognitive health." (The Stanford study is in the journal *Translational Psychiatry*.)

In simple language, BDNF truly is Miracle-Gro for the brain. It's the real deal for brain function, and a modest amount of regular exercise will keep it in abundant supply.

* * *

A personal—and unscientific—testimonial would seem to be in order. Short bouts of exercise stimulate my brain; no question about it. Some of my best thinking is done during the short walks (~ 10 minutes) I take periodically during the day.

These walks help me connect the dots, so to speak, putting related ideas together. Within the first block or so, solutions regularly start coming to me. New words or phrases or better

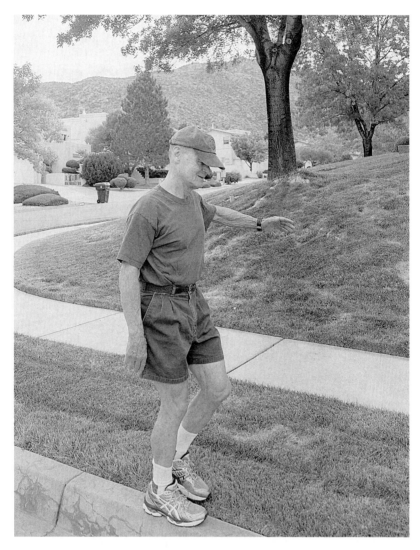

Some of my best thinking is done during the short walks I take during the day. *Photo by Laszlo Bencze*

ways to express myself or missing elements pop up, often when I'm thinking about something else.

The same thing happens to me during the night—possibly aided by a lifetime of exercise—usually after 4 or 5 hours of sleep. I drive Carol crazy turning the light on and off writing notes to myself. (If I don't write it down, I have trouble going back to sleep.)

The creative process is miraculous—and accessible to just

about everyone. Nothing sparks it like exercise. Sleep is close. Coffee is barely in the ballpark.

*   *   *

For centuries, we've believed that lifestyle affects lifespan, for good or ill, but precisely how and why have for the most part remained matters of conjecture. *Biomarkers* was perhaps the first book to provide a definitive list of the factors associated with aging that can be changed for the better through lifestyle—and back it up with facts. Drs. Evans and Rosenberg explained in detail how exercise improves each of their signposts of aging.

Exercise is the number one arrow in our quiver of life expanding tools. Each one of us has the power to put it to work. Exercise is the bargain of bargains; the primary cost is sweat equity. Exercise is our number one take-charge tool.

Science is not only proving that exercise works, it is telling us how and why.

Chapter Six
Exercise and Aging

New Pattern of Aging

Two Harvard scientists did a study of the world's fastest growing age group, people over 100, and gave us a new and more positive picture of living long.

In *Living To 100* (Basic books, 1999), Thomas T. Perls, M.D., and Margery Hutter Silver, Ed.D., director and associate director of the New England Centenarian Study, tell us what it's like to live to 100 or more and what we can learn from people who've done it.

In a survey, 63 percent said they didn't want to live to be 100, mostly because of worries about declining health and loss of mental faculties. After studying more than one hundred centenarians, interviewing them in their homes, scrutinizing their family trees, and assessing their physical and mental health, Perls and Silver uncovered a new pattern of aging never recognized before, a pattern that may give those surveyed reason to think anew. Contrary to popular perception and until recently the expectations of most geriatricians, people over 100—about 1 in 4,400 Americans, about three times as many as there were in 1980—are a surprisingly sprightly group.

The assumption that age and disease go hand in hand, Perls and Silver found, is wrong. Older does not necessarily mean sicker. In fact, according to these specialists, most centenarians are able to delay illness to a short period at the very end of their life. Perls and Silver say that compressed morbidity seems to be a characteristic of the very old. Long painful declines are seen more in people who die late in middle age. Most centenarians seem to have found a way to maximize the healthy portion of their very long lives.

My grandmother died at home, without spending a single day in a nursing home or a hospital during her final years. I visited her unannounced many times—she lived a few blocks from my parents—and she was always beautifully dressed and happy to see me. It came as a surprise to everyone when she passed away in her sleep—at 98.

I never knew her to do any formal exercise, but she always cleaned her own house; it was not unusual to find her on her knees scrubbing her kitchen floor. She stayed trim and watched the 10 o'clock news every night before going to bed.

Jack LaLanne, who died in 2011, at 96, was another example of the new pattern of aging. As I wrote at the time, he celebrated his 95th birthday with a 'knock-your-socks-off' autobiographical

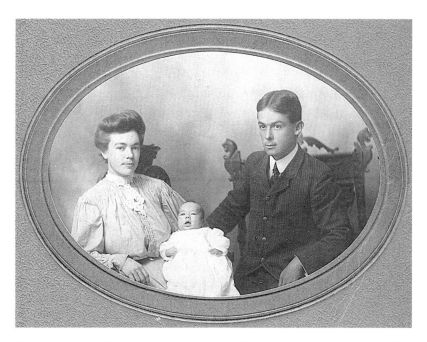

This treasured family photo, taken in 1906, shows my grandmother and grandfather, and my father as a baby. *Photo by Pennington Davis*

overview of his life full of wisdom for all ages. I saw him on Fox News during the last year of his life, and he was firing on all cylinders. According to reports from his family, he was only ill for a short time before his death. He died at home from respiratory failure due to pneumonia. Wanting to go out on his own terms, he refused to be hospitalized.

Like those studied by Perls and Silver, Jack barely missed a beat until a brief period immediately before death.

How do the very old manage to age so well? How can the rest of us put the centenarians' longevity lessons to work in our lives?

It helps to have good genes, of course. If one or more of your parents, grandparents or perhaps an aunt or uncle lived to extreme old age in good health, that improves your odds—but it's not essential.

Perls and Silver say the majority of us have strong enough longevity genes to live to age 85 or so, and we can compress the time that we're sick to the very end of our lives. The key is to make the best of the genes we have. "People who take appropriate preventative steps may add as many as ten quality years to that," say the authors. "People who fail to heed the messages of preventive medicine may subtract substantial years from their lives." In large measure it's up to us.

Carol and I used the "Life Expectancy Calculator" in the book to see how we're doing. Although I picked up a few years by having a grandmother and two aunts who reached their late 90s in good health, Carol used the female advantage to edge me out with a life expectancy of 99.1 years to my 96.6.

*   *   *

Fitness is one of the primary controllable factors on the road to a long and healthy life.

Live Fit, Live Long

The more fit you are the longer you are likely to live.

"As you increase your ability to exercise—increase your fitness—you are decreasing in a step-wise fashion the risk of death," Peter Kokkinos, MD, lead researcher in a recent study, told *HealthDay News*.

Become more fit and live longer. That is the basic conclusion of a study released January 23, 2008, in the online edition of *Circulation*, the journal of the American Heart Association. "The major finding is that for all sorts of people, as one increases his exercise capacity based on an exercise treadmill test, there is an inverse drop [in death risk] in a dose response fashion," Dr. Kokkinos told *Heartwire*, a professional news service of WebMD. In short, the more fit you are the less likely you are to die. This happens in a direct, one-for-one manner—fitness up, mortality down.

We've known for a long time that exercise can dramatically prolong life. What makes this study special is its size and diversity. The study was government sponsored and the largest of its kind. Earlier studies involved mostly white subjects from higher socioeconomic classes.

Kokkinos and his colleagues followed 15,660 black and white male veterans for an average of 7.5 years after completion of a treadmill test to measure their exercise capacity. The participants ranged in age from 47 to 71 (mean age 59); they were more than 40% black. Some had cardiovascular disease and some didn't. One third were obese.

The men were divided into four fitness categories based on their treadmill performance in METS or metabolic equivalents. One MET is the normal oxygen uptake when at rest.

Results were as follows:

1) Exercise capacity was the strongest predictor of death; for both black and white men, fitness level was more powerful than age, cardiovascular risk factors, blood pressure or body mass index in predicting the risk of death.

2) Risk of death was reduced by an average of 13% for every 1-MET increase in exercise capacity; the mortality reduction per MET was 14% for blacks and 12% for whites.

3) The risk of death went down with each step up in fitness category; those classified as moderately fit (5 to 7 METS) had a 20% lower risk of death compared to low-fit men (<5 METS). High-fit men (7.1 to 10 METS) had a 50% lower risk, and those with very high fitness reduced their risk of dying by 70%. In short, the odds of survival for the fittest men were more than three times better than for the least fit men.

What about women? "Although we don't know from this research that this applies to women as well, there's no reason to suspect that it wouldn't," Alice Lichtenstein, director of the Cardiovascular Nutrition Lab at Tufts University, told *Health-Day News*.

The practice tip for physicians, according to the researchers, is to pay as much attention to a patient's fitness as to other major risk factors, such as age, cardiovascular risk factors, and body weight.

"Everyone needs to get involved to get this nation going again, because we are the fattest nation, the most sedentary nation in the world," Dr. Kokkinos told *Heartwire*. "We could do something like walking for thirty minutes a day and reap major benefits," he added.

The 2007 guidelines from the American College of Sports Medicine and the American Heart Associate give specific suggestions on what else you can do to become more fit.

For the average healthy adult, the minimum requirement is moderate intensity exercise (brisk walking) for 30 minutes five days a week or vigorous exercise (running, basketball, singles tennis) for 20 minutes three days a week. You can also mix it up by combining moderate and intense exercise. For example, walk for 30 minutes twice a week and jog for 20 minutes on two other days. Working out more, or harder, will increase the benefits. (We'll talk about the advantages of more intense exercise later in this chapter.)

If you're pressed for time—or not inclined to jog—interval

training is an equally effective, perhaps more effective, option. (See Chapter 3)

Strength training (8 to 10 different exercises) two or three times a week is recommended to prevent loss of muscle and bone, and make daily activities easier. (More on strength training below)

Stretching and balancing exercises are also recommended whenever you exercise. This is especially important for those over 65, but good advice for young people as well.

Any amount of exercise at any intensity is better than none, of course. The key is to do something most days, and add things you enjoy as your fitness improves. Most people do best with a variety of activities to keep them interested and motivated.

*   *   *

Athletes are proving the fitness-enhancing value of challenging yourself throughout life.

Athletes Winning Over Age

Not long ago it was "time to hang it up" when an athlete hit 40. You were definitely over the hill at 50. Now it's 75—and maybe later.

That's my take on a study published March, 2008, in the *American Journal of Sports Medicine*. It is essentially what Vonda J. Wright, MD, and Brett C. Perricelli, MD, professors of orthopedics at the University of Pittsburgh, found after analyzing performance times at the 2001 National Senior Olympic Games (age 50 to 85), and comparing the results with those of American track and field record holders.

Importantly, these results are for people who are in serious training, not the average Joe or Jane jogging on the street—and certainly not the average sedentary American. The people in this study were competing and trying to improve; some continued training as they got older and others started competing in middle age.

Let's look at what the study found, and then talk about how to do as well, or perhaps better.

Wright and Perricelli found that year-to-year performance declined after 50, but at a rate that was barely noticeable until about 75, when the decline became undeniable. These figures are averages, of course; some did better and some worse. Remember, these are competing athletes.

Times for men and women, sprinters (100-400m) and distance runners (1500-10,000m), were analyzed and plotted, from ages 50 to 85 for participants in the 2001 Games, and 30 to 85 for the American record holders. The actual numbers are a statistician's delight, but mind numbing for most of us. The following averages provide a good overview of the results.

For Senior Games winners, the average yearly percentage increase in times (performance decline), from 50 to 85, for all track distances, was 3.44% for men and 3.36% for women. Most of the decline, however, took place in the last 10 years, from 75 to 85. For American record holders, the average yearly decline was less: 1.9% for men, and 3.31% for women. Again, most of the decline took place after 75.

Men did better than women after 75. Among men, the record holders did best after 75. Among women, Senior Olympic Games winners prevailed. Men record holders declined at one half the rate of Games participants after 75, 4.1% vs. 7.86%. On the other hand, female winners at the Games did better than the record holders; Games winners declined 7.36% compared to 10.29% for American record holders.

Pretty clearly, more is going on here than aging. It's a safe bet that the American record holders were better trained than Games participants, and over-75 men may have been more motivated than the over-75 women. Men probably outnumbered the women too.

Training and motivation, along with age, were probably factors. It's telling I believe, that variability among the top 8 winning times increased markedly with advancing age. The gap between top competitors widened—perhaps along with motivation and other circumstances beyond age—some did a lot better than others.

Who knows what's really possible as we age?

As Dr. Bruce Reider observed in an editorial accompanying the study, these champion athletes are by definition "outliers," ahead of the crowd. Even among elites, however, there are variations. Dr. Reider is optimistic about future prospects. "Although age-related decline in our athletic patients may be inevitable," he writes, "studies have shown that continued or renewed training can mitigate its progression, even in nonagenarians [90 to 100 year-olds]."

Let's look at training to improve strength and endurance.

This study is only the first step in understanding the relationship between age and performance. The next question is: How

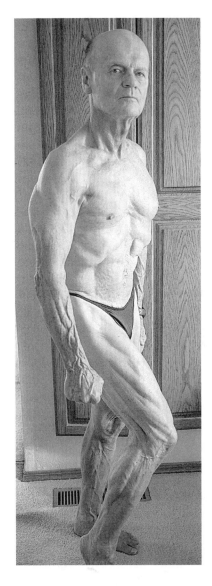

At 75, I'm at the usual point of rapid decline. Time will tell. I intend to
keep training hard and looking for
ways to improve.

Photo by Laszlo Bencze

can athletes and nonathletes do better? What's the best way of
preserving and improving muscle strength and aerobic capacity?

Drs. Wright and Perricelli point the way in the "Discussion"
portion of the study.

"Muscle power is lost at a greater rate than endurance capacity," they observe, "3.5% versus 1.8% per year." That makes
strength training a top priority as we age.

Sound familiar? (We began talking about this in Chapter 1.)

A decrease in the size and number of muscle fibers with age

is a significant issue; fast-twitch fibers are particularly vulnerable. "Individual fibers shrink approximately 30% between the ages of 20 and 80," the doctors relate. "Paralleling the decline in performance seen in the study, muscle fiber number declines modestly until the age of 50 years, and increases more rapidly thereafter." The nerves that activate muscle cells also degenerate, which adds to the problem. "Muscle cells require stimulation from motor nerve cells to live, and without it, they too atrophy," the doctors explain. Use it or lose it.

Aerobic exercise alone will not maintain muscle mass, said Wright and Perricelli. "Only strength-trained seniors [have] muscle mass and composition similar to that of young controls," they report.

"All these factors point to the critical need for resistance training after the age of 50 years for maintenance of muscle strength," the doctors concluded.

Aerobic or endurance capacity must not be neglected, of course. As we saw in Chapter 4, strength training also builds— or helps maintain—aerobic capacity.

"Reductions in VO2max are believed to be the primary reason for a decline in functional endurance with aging," the researchers stated. The answer is "intense habitual exercise," which maintains cardiac output. "As training intensity declines, so does the VO2max," the doctors wrote.

High-intensity aerobics is the key, not long, slow endurance training. Break out of the "aerobic zone." Challenge your maximum heart rate. Again, use it or lose it.

* * *

New York Times fitness writer Gina Kolata confirmed the primacy of hard, brief training in her January 31, 2008, column "Staying a Step Ahead of Aging."

Kolata went to Steven Hawkins, an exercise physiologist at the University of Southern California, for guidance. "When you have to choose between hard and often, choose hard," he told her. "High performance is really determined more by intensity than volume," he added. "When you're older, something has to give. You can't have both so you have to cut back on the volume. You need more rest days."

Hawkins practices what he preaches. "I run a couple of times a week and I try to make it as fast as I can," he told Kolata.

That's it. Hard weights. Intense aerobics. Rest.

That threesome will keep you going strong longer than you ever dreamed possible.

(Check with your doctor if you're out of shape or have health problems.)

* * *

Now, we'll look at two eye-opening studies showing the power of exercise to prevent or overcome the devastating effects of aging. The first study involves mice, and the second humans. Both are striking examples of the power of exercise.

Exercise Proves Amazing Rejuvenator

"While the exercised mice scampered and scurried about their cages, the aging non-runners huddled in a corner, barely moving," Sharon Kirkey, writing in the *Montreal Gazette* (February 22, 2011), captured the breath-taking imagery of this study.

Exercise is the closest thing we're likely to find to the proverbial Fountain of Youth. Ask Mark Tarnopolsky, professor of pediatrics and medicine at McMaster University. He put fast-aging mice on a running program—with phenomenal results. Exercise rejuvenated virtually every tissue and organ in their bodies, including mitochondria, muscle mass, brain, heart, and gonads.

Tarnopolsky's study is grounded in the mitochondrial theory of aging. The mice used were ideally suited to test the hypothesis—and the power of exercise.

Researchers are increasingly seeing aging as a mitochondrial disease. Defective mitochondria appear as we get older, robbing us of endurance, strength, and function. Mitochondria combine oxygen and nutrients to create fuel for virtually every cell in the body. When mitochondria go bad, cells all over the body begin to wither and die.

Tarnopolsky and colleagues used mice lacking the primary mitochondria repair mechanism, which caused them to begin aging rapidly at about three months, the human equivalent of 20 years. By the time they reached eight months (60 for humans), they were old, inside and out. All were dead before reaching one year. All, that is, but the runners.

The mice were genetically engineered to age rapidly due to defective mitochondrial polymerase gamma (PolG), which disrupts the repair of mitochondria. The engineered animals, called *PolG Mice*, had previously provided the "first direct cause-and-effect evidence" that dysfunctional mitochondria result in premature aging and related pathologies, Tarnopolsky and colleagues explained in their report.

Mitochondria are unique in that they have their own DNA. Accumulated damage to the mitochondrial DNA leads to an energy crisis which results in a progressive decline in tissue and organ function. Without a repair mechanism, these mice were targeted for premature aging. Tarnopolsky's sedentary mice deteriorated as expected, but not their fellow mutants that began running at three months.

The mice ran on a wheel for 45 minutes three times a week, at about 15 minutes per mile. "It was about like a person running a 50- or 55-minute 10K," principal investigator Tarnopolsky related. (10K is 6.2 miles.) The mice continued running for five months.

The mice that ran remained youthful and healthy, while their sedentary peers were balding, graying, shrinking, and losing interest in the opposite sex. The runners had full pelts and no graying. They maintained their muscle mass and brain volume. Their gonads and ovaries were normal, along with their hearts.

"Not only did the treadmill-running mice look as sleek-coated, bright-eyed, and bushy-tailed as wild mice, but the researchers also saw huge recovery in age-related damage to practically every tissue they could analyze," The *Montreal Gazette* reported.

"Every part of the body was protected by exercise," Tarnopolsky reported enthusiastically. "I think that exercise is the most potent anti-aging therapy available today or likely forever."
It's not clear just how exercise changed the aging process of these mice. What is clear is that exercise stimulated mitochondria by some mechanism outside the normal pathway, which didn't exist for these mutant mice.

The researchers offered several theories. One is that exercise promoted regeneration of healthy mitochondria not affected by defective polymerase. In addition, they speculated that endurance exercise stimulated release of metabolites that "may promote organ cross-talk, resulting in systemic mitochondrial biogenesis and multisystem rejuvenation. These adaptations may [dilute] the pathological effects of mitochondrial DNA point mutations incurred systemically in PolG mice."

Dr. Tarnopolsky is currently overseeing experiments to uncover the precise mechanisms involved. But for now, he says, the lesson of this experiment and many others like it is unambiguous: "Exercise alters the course of aging."

"Others have tried to treat these animals with exercise pill drugs and have even tried to reduce their caloric intake, a strategy felt to be most effective for slowing aging, and those were met with limited success," Tarnopolsky related.

Research also has a lighter side.

While many were impressed that the active mice kept their hair, it may take more to move the younger crowd. Dr. Tarnopolsky confided to *New York Times* writer Gretchen Reynolds that his younger graduate students were most interested in the animal's robust gonads. "I think they all exercise now," he said.

Adding a more serious note, Dr. Tarnopolsky told *The New York Times* that aerobic exercise is not the only form of exercise that alters aging. Studies of older humans have shown that weightlifting can also improve mitochondrial health, he noted to Gretchen Reynolds.

If you haven't been exercising, walking is a good place to start. "Anything is better than nothing," Tarnopolsky counseled.

(The Tarnopolsky team study was published on February 21, 2011, in the journal *Proceedings of the National Academy of Sciences.*)

* * *

Let's move on to the study involving humans, which is, perhaps, even more persuasive than the mouse study. Exercise was found to be far more important than age in determining fitness and health.

Exercise Overcomes 30 Years of Aging

Norwegian researchers have produced what may be the most important evidence so far of the power of exercise to combat the effects of aging.

They used the world's largest fitness database to directly measure the relationship between fitness and various assessments of overall health. Stian Thoresen Aspense was awarded his PhD for his study of 4631 healthy men and women of all ages who underwent extensive laboratory examination to measure peak fitness and a troublesome cluster of risk factors that dispose people to diabetes, stroke, and heart problems. Participants were also given an activity index score, based on exercise frequency, duration, and intensity.

The researchers postulated at the beginning of the study that fitness may be the single best predictor of cardiovascular and other death rates.

Other studies have come to similar conclusions, but they used indirect measurements of fitness or were based on small populations. Aspense, principle investigator Dr. Ulrik Wisloff, and colleagues used direct measurement of VO2peak to assess the association between fitness, aging, and risk factors. "These data represent the largest reference material of objectively measured VO2peak in healthy men and women 20-90 years," the researchers wrote.

Science Daily tells us that the underpinnings of the Aspense-Wisloff research go back to a 1965 study conducted in Dallas, Texas, which highlighted the devastating effect of inactivity. *Science Daily* called it "one of the most famous fitness studies of all time." The Dallas researchers selected five healthy 20-year-olds to spend three weeks in bed. Predictably, they lost fitness—VO2max dropped by a huge 27 percent. The biggest surprise, however, came 30 years later, when researchers retested the same men.

"Time had not been so charitable to these men," *Science Daily* wrote. Their body fat had doubled—they'd gained over 50 pounds on average—and they were far from fit. Their peak oxygen uptake, however, had dropped by only 11 percent as compared to their 20-year-old healthy selves.

Thirty years of aging decreased their fitness less than half as much as three weeks in bed!

The Norwegian researchers went beyond the Dallas findings. They reversed the process—substituting activity for inactivity—and showed that exercise can stop the decline in fitness that typically comes with aging. They found that fit 50-year olds can be every bit as fit as 20-year olds who don't exercise. "VO2peak in inactive participants aged 20-29 was nearly identical with that of highly active participants 50-59 years," the Aspense-Wisloff team reported.

In short, exercise stopped the normal decline of fitness in its tracks.

What form of exercise—how much and how hard—worked best?

When the Norwegian researchers looked at the importance of intensity versus duration, intensity was found to be far more important than duration in determining peak fitness levels. (They had earlier confirmed that high-intensity interval training is a quick and effective way to increase overall fitness.)

Importantly, Aspense-Wisloff et al also examined the relationship between fitness and risk factors. They found that both men and women benefited substantially healthwise from above average fitness levels.

"Women below median VO2peak were five times and men below median were eight times more likely to have a cluster of cardiovascular risk factors compared to those in the highest quartile of VO2peak," Aspense-Wisloff et al wrote. "Each 5 [oxygen processing units] lower VO2peak corresponded to about 56% higher odds of cardiovascular risk factor clustering."

Clearly, exercise pays big dividends in health as well as fitness—the fitter you are the healthier you are likely to be.

"Physical condition is the most important factor in describing an individual's overall health, almost like a report card," Stian Thoresen Aspense told *Science Daily*.

The Aspense-Wisloff study was reported in the August, 2011, issue of the journal *Medicine & Science in Sports & Exercise*.

* * *

Keep in mind that these findings are statistical averages. Wonderful as they are, enthusiastic lifetime trainers are likely to benefit even more. You'll see how much more in the next section, where I'll tell you about the main findings of a professor who has methodically researched and written a book about the best forms of exercise to keep us young and fit. We've touched on many of the professor's points, but it's helpful—and motivating—to have a detailed and clear explanation of how exercise combats aging.

Bending the Aging Curve

Joseph F. Signorile, PhD, is a highly regarded professor of exercise physiology at the University of Miami in Coral Gables, Florida, and co-author (with Arthur Agatston, MD) of *The South Beach Diet Super Charged* (Rodale, 2008). Dr. Signorile makes the case for interval training in both books, but goes far beyond that in his new book. He provides a complete exercise guide for making us younger, stronger, fitter, and healthier.

Dr. Signorile's book, *Bending the Aging Curve*, was published by Human Kinetics in 2011.

Signorile uses a wonderfully apt metaphor to capsulize his message. He recalls the advertising slogan of the Castrol oil company that you could spend a few dollars to change your oil now or you could spend a few thousand dollars later to change your engine. It's the corporate version of *an ounce of prevention or a pound of cure*. "Somewhere along the way we have lost sight of this simple concept in our health care system," Signorile wrote. "Rather than using simple tools such as exercise and

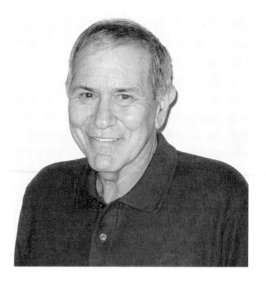

Dr. Signorile has written over 50 refereed articles and book chapters and presented at countless national and international scientific and industry meetings. *Photo courtesy of Signorile*

diet to help reduce the negative effects of aging, we allow physical declines to occur and then address them with prescription drugs, assistive devices, and rehabilitation."

Why wait until you need a new engine—or a new body—when you can simply change your oil? Listen to Professor Signorile. Take charge now.

Bending the Aging Curve includes many tables and graphs, but the one that sums up the message best is a graph showing the neuromuscular aging curves for the untrained person, for the person who starts exercising at about 40, and finally the trajectory of men and women who have been exercising their entire life. The differences are stunning.

The loss of neuromuscular function for untrained individuals begins in earnest at about 40 and drops more and more rapidly with each passing decade; the decline is exponential. The person who begins exercising at 40 shows a relatively flat curve until about 60, and then begins a slow decline. The lifelong exerciser, however, soars above the others at every decade of life. The lifelong exerciser has a curve that begins at a much higher level than the other two—and stays there. The inevitable decline that does occur leaves the 75-year-old lifelong exerciser at a level equivalent to an untrained person at 20. At 90, the lifelong trainer is at a level equivalent to an untrained person 30 years younger.

If that doesn't make you want to exercise, nothing will.

Professor Signorile covers body composition, testing, flexibility, bone density, muscular strength and endurance, cardiovascular fitness, periodization, and functional training for the activities of daily living. (I told you it's a complete exercise guide.) We can't cover all that here, but we can relate a few of the salient points.

Let's start with a look at the aging curves of slow twitch and fast twitch muscle fibers, which fare quite differently for people who exercise and those who don't, especially after the age of 50. It's no secret that muscle size and strength drop rapidly after the age of 50. When we understand the physiology of muscle fibers, however, it becomes apparent that the big drop isn't inevitable; it can be countered or reversed.

As noted earlier, the loss of muscle size that occurs as we age is called *sarcopenia*, taken from Greek meaning "abnormal reduction" or "deficiency." Sarcopenia occurs for two reasons. First, individual muscle cells (fibers) shrink and eventually die. Because muscle fibers are bundled together, when individual fibers shrink, the whole bundle loses size. In addition, every muscle fiber has a nerve, called a *motor nerve*, which innervates it. For efficiency, motor units branch out and control many muscle fibers (100 to 10,000). The motor nerve and the fibers it controls are called a *motor unit*.

"As we age, our motor nerves and their associated muscle fibers die off at an ever increasing rate," Signorile explains. "A small percentage of these fibers are rescued by neighboring motor units, but the number of living fibers still drops exponentially...The bottom line is that as we age we not only have smaller but also fewer muscle fibers."

Fiber type also plays a major role in muscle size. Slow-twitch fibers are small, and fast-twitch fibers are large. The slow-twitch fibers are the endurance fibers, which predominate in marathon runners and other endurance athletes. Fast-twitch fibers are the strength fibers, which rule the roost in sprinters, weight lifters, and other strength athletes. They are strong, but fatigue rapidly. Most of us are born with a roughly equal balance of slow/small and fast/large fibers.

"*As we age, the motor units that we lose are mainly the fast-twitch variety,*" Signorile wrote. (My emphasis) "The slow-twitch fibers show practically no change." This phenomenon is due, in part, to the rescue process mentioned earlier. "During the rescue process, slow-twitch motor units rescue fast-twitch fibers and change them into slow-twitch fibers. So the cost of rescuing a few fibers is that the aging muscle shows a predominance of slow-twitch fibers."

Signorile uses another graph to show the pattern of change in fast and slow twitch muscle fibers as we age. This one, however, can be described in a few words. The curve of the slow-twitch fibers over time is no curve at all; it's flat, showing essentially the same number of slow fibers at 60 and 90. On the other hand, the fast-fiber curve drops rapidly from 60 to 90.

In short, the loss of muscle size with age is virtually all due to shrinkage and death of fast-twitch fibers. Translated to the activities of everyday life, this means the untrained person becomes slower and weaker with age. Independence suffers over time.

It's a dismal picture, but all is not lost. Far from it. We can keep our fast-twitch fibers alive and well with resistance training. Signorile is a big booster of resistance training. His chapter on the subject is the longest in book, at 76 pages. Again, we can only cover a few of the most important points here.

How many people are affected by sarcopenia? "A lot," says Signorile. "It has been estimated that from the age of 60 to 80 the prevalence of sarcopenia in the general population progresses from 15% to 32% for men and 23% to 36% for women. After the age of 80 these values increase to 51% for women and 55% for men."

It's a big problem.

Reduced physical activity is the main culprit. Resistance training is the best antidote. "Resistance training has been shown to positively affect neurological, hormonal, and mechanical factors associated with muscle maintenance and growth," Signorile wrote. "You could fill up a small warehouse with articles touting the benefits of resistance exercise in reducing sarcopenia and its impact on independence, falls, and mobility."

Front and center is the effect on the fast-twitch muscle fibers, the type 2 fibers, which are most dramatically affected by the aging process. Resistance training increases the size of the type 2 fibers and the ability of the motor nerves to recruit those fibers. Resistance training also increases the ability of the fast fibers to repair themselves, thus reaching higher levels of hypertrophy.

On the biochemical side, resistance training increases levels of testosterone and growth hormone. What's more, it increases blood glucose utilization and ATP production and recycling. (ATP stands for *adenosine triphosphate*, the chemical source of energy for muscle action. It serves to store energy in muscles.)

There are more benefits, but those are some of the most transparent.

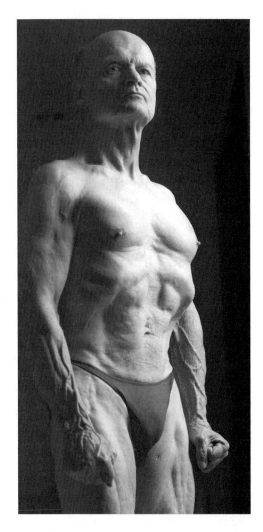

You don't have to lose muscle mass as you age. Reduced physical activity is the main culprit. Resistance training is the best antidote.

Photo by Laszlo Bencze

Now, let's move on to cardiovascular fitness and aging.

The most common measure of cardiovascular capacity is maximal oxygen uptake, or VO2max. VO2max is a measure of the maximal rate at which your body can use oxygen, or simply your aerobic power. As in the case of neuromuscular function, an exponential drop in maximal aerobic power occurs with age. Men and women decline at essentially the same rate, with men having marginally higher VO2max throughout life.

Again, it doesn't have to be that way.

"Researchers who examine training protocols to increase aerobic capacity consistently report that high-intensity exercise produces greater improvement in VO2max than low- or moderate-intensity exercise produce," Dr. Signorile wrote. If improving aerobic power is the goal, "intensity is the name of the game."

Interval training is the most effective and efficient form of high-intensity cardiovascular training—for old and young alike. "If increasing aerobic capacity, reducing high blood pressure, or weight loss (especially around the waistline) is the goal, then interval training is one of the most effective tools you possess to reach that goal," Signorile wrote.

Dr. Signorile offered the following study as evidence of the superiority of interval training for older individuals.

"One study compared moderate-intensity continuous training (70% peak HR) with aerobic interval training (95% peak HR) performed three times per week for 12 weeks," Signorile wrote. "The subjects were 27 postinfarction heart failure patients and the average age was 75.7 years. *VO2 peak increased more than three times as much with the interval training than it did with the moderate continuous training.*" (Emphasis mine)

What's more, Signorile added, only interval training improved "the filling and emptying capacity of the heart" and the ability of the arteries to accommodate increased blood flow.

What's the most efficient interval training work/rest ratio to improve the cardiovascular system?

Signorile responded, "The winner is…the old 2:1 standby composed of 20 seconds of work and 10 seconds of recovery." (Sound familiar? We used this quote in Chapter 3.)

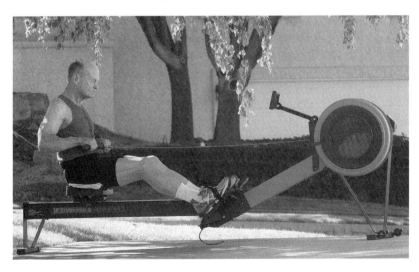

If building and maintaining aerobic power is the goal, intensity is the name of the game. *Photo by Laszlo Bencze*

It describes the original Tabata protocol.

That, however, doesn't mean that Dr. Signorile recommended only one ratio. He wisely suggested a varied approach to interval training. "This is not to say that a work-recovery duty cycle of 20 seconds to 10 seconds is the panacea of cardiovascular training. In fact, the best idea is to use a diverse mix of work-recovery cycles…"

In addition to work-recovery ratio, other variables are the length of the work cycle, intensity, and number of work-recovery cycles. The options are almost limitless.

Dr. Signorile listed several practical guidelines to keep in mind when planning intervals:

"Short work cycles (10 to 20s) allow the highest intensity, while short rest periods (20 to 40s) limit recovery between reps. Moderately-short work cycles (30s) allow for fairly high intensity, and somewhat longer recovery periods (60s) allow more complete recovery. Longer work cycles (60s) require the most difficult mix of work and recovery (60 to 120s), perhaps too difficult to be feasible for non-athletes. Finally, very long work (2 to 5 min) and recovery (4 to 10 min) cycles are impractical, and make it more beneficial to simply do steady state exercise."

*   *   *

My suggestion is to make intervals as hard as you can tolerate without killing motivation—hard but not too hard.

As in the case of resistance training, variation is the key to long term success in cardiovascular training. Change keeps you motivated and gives your body (and your mind) an opportunity to adapt and grow stronger and fitter.

Signorile provided details on a wide range of aerobic and resistance training options, including volume resistance training and steady state aerobic training. If you want chapter and verse on strength and cardiovascular training and design—and much more—Dr. Signorile's *Bending the Aging Curve* (Human Kinetics, 2011) is the book for you.

Train regularly—strength and aerobic. Flatten your aging curve. If you haven't already, start now—and don't stop.

*   *   *

Now, let's talk about a recently-discovered risk factor. It came as a surprise to many of us who work out regularly—and didn't know we had a problem. The risks are eye opening—and the many bonuses that come from addressing the problem are reassuring.

Chapter Seven
Too Much Sitting

Too Much Sitting Is Risky—
Even for People Who Train

"Just sitting as most people do [between workouts] is health detrimental," Dr. Richard Winett wrote in an e-mail. I was soon to learn that he was onto something big—a brand new risk factor. (Professor Winett spends many of his waking hours working at a computer, so it was important news for both of us.)

"Sedentary pursuits represent a *unique aspect of human behavior* and should not be viewed as simply the extreme low end of the physical activity continuum," Canadian researcher Peter T. Katzmarzyk, PhD, and colleagues wrote in a 2009 study called to my attention by Winett. (We'll discuss the study below)

Man is apparently the only animal to figure out how to survive sitting down most of the time.

How much time do you spend riding in a car, working at a desk, eating at a table, playing video games, using a computer, watching TV, or engaged in other sedentary pursuits? Think about it. It may be a problem. Even if you exercise regularly.

In the '60s, I remember reading in *Strength & Health* that Dr. Terry Todd, arguably the best power lifter in the world at the time and editor of the magazine, was working from bed to enhance recovery between his brutal workouts. In my mind's eye, I can still see the photo of 300-pounds plus Todd with papers spread all over his bed. The plan must not have panned out very well, because I never read or heard any more about it.

Todd downsized himself a few years later, and has never regained the weight. He kept lifting and continues to stay active to this day. He was wiser than anyone knew.

I've long maintained that walking between workouts burns extra calories and helps speed recovery. Turns out that's not the half of it.

Neville Owen (School of Population Health, University of Queensland, Brisbane, Australia) and two colleagues warned in the *British Journal of Sports Medicine* (2009) that the widely recommended 30 minutes of moderate to vigorous activity 3 to 5 days a week may not alone be sufficient. "Recent evidence underlines the importance of also focusing on sedentary behaviors—the high volume of time that adults spend sitting in their remaining 'non-exercising' waking hours," they wrote.

Calling too much sitting a *new field* of concern, they continued: "Our recent body of work has identified sedentary behavior (time spent sitting) as a novel and potentially important risk

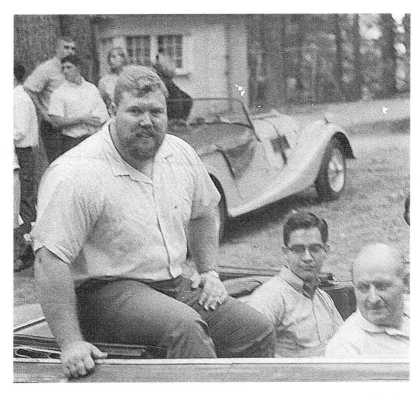

This historic photo, taken in 1965, shows Terry Todd the day after he won the first official Senior National Powerlifting Championship. He was at or near his highest bodyweight—335. Not only was he wise enough to drop weight after his glory days in lifting, he went on to become a professor at the University of Texas (Austin) where he is now the Director of the Stark Center for Physical Culture and Sports.

Photo courtesy of Dr. Todd

factor for development of chronic disease...There may be significant metabolic and health effects from prolonged sitting."

The researchers said that most adults spend more than half of their waking hours in sedentary activities (mostly sitting), with the remainder of the time spent in light intensity activities (standing with some movement); "only about 4.5% of the day is spent in moderate to vigorous physical activity."

Owen and co-authors said we need to begin thinking about ways to break periods of prolonged sitting. "Commonsense might suggest that it may be prudent to try to minimize prolonged sitting with 5 minute breaks every hour," they wrote.

A number of studies have uncovered specific health risks involved in too much inactivity. Let's look at two called to my attention by Dr. Winett, starting with the study alluded to earlier. Peter T. Katzmarzyk, PhD, and colleagues from Canada and the U.S. followed 17,013 Canadian men and women 18-90 years of age for an average of 12 years, looking into the relationship between sitting time and deaths from all causes. Their report appeared in *Medicine & Science in Sports & Exercise* (2009).

Subjects were grouped based on the portion of the day spent sitting (almost none, one fourth, half, three fourths, and almost all day). Participants were also classified as active or inactive based on current minimum physical activity recommendations.

What they found is a wake-up call, especially to those complying with recommended exercise guidelines.

They found a progressively higher rate of mortality as sitting time increased. For example, participants who spent three fourths of their day sitting were 36% to 47% more likely to die than those who spent only one fourth of the day sitting. Tellingly, it didn't make any difference whether subjects were otherwise active or inactive; death rates were essentially the same for those who exercised regularly and those who didn't exercise.

"This is an important observation," the researchers wrote in the Discussion portion of the report, "because it suggests that high amounts of sitting cannot be compensated for with occasional leisure time physical activity even if the amount exceeds the current minimum physical activity recommendations."

In other words, regular workouts (90 minutes or five hours a week) do not allow us to sit around without consequences.

The next study, reported in the *Scandinavian Journal of Medicine and Science in Sports* (2008), highlighted two ways that staying active between workouts may help.

M. Hamer and A. Steptoe (Department of Epidemiology and Public Health, University College, London) examined the impact of walking on inflammation and hemostasis (sluggishness of blood flow), separate and apart from vigorous physical activity.

The participants (107 men and 78 women, age 45 to 59) were asked how many minutes they walk each week and how often they engage in vigorous activities, such as running, that make them feel out of breath.

Walking 30 minutes or more a day was found to be significantly associated with lower inflammation and hemostatic markers. Vigorous activity was associated with lower levels of hemostatic markers, but not lower inflammatory markers.

Walking appeared to lower both markers, with the positive effect on inflammation being unique. Walking lowered inflammation, but vigorous exercise did not. Both walking and vigorous exercise improved blood flow.

*　*　*

It's no surprise that vigorous exercise increases inflammation, at least temporarily. Inflammation is part of the normal healing process. Walking helps to moderate the inflammation caused by vigorous exercise. The two forms of exercise complement one another. In my book *Challenge Yourself*, I called the combination of high-intensity aerobics and low-intensity walking "A Barbell Aerobics Strategy," high intensity on one end of the barbell and low intensity on the other end. It works wonderfully well.

Those who engage in vigorous exercise—weights and aerobics—would be well advised to walk or engage in some other form of mild physical activity on most days.

*　*　*

Happily, researchers and others are helping us fight back and win the war against inactivity.

Fight Back Against Too Much Sitting

Dr. James Levine, a researcher at the Mayo Clinic in Rochester, MN, and a leader in the fast emerging field of inactivity studies, calls too much sitting is "a lethal activity." Thanks to Levine and others like him, the field is exploding with new findings and ways to fight back.

What happens when we sit?

"The muscles go as silent as those of a dead horse," explained Marc Hamilton, an inactivity researcher at Pennington Biomedical Research Center in Louisiana. That leads to a cascade of harmful metabolic effects. Your calorie burn rate immediately plunges to about one per minute, a third of what it would be if you got up and walked around, according to Hamilton.

Hamilton's research has shown that rats forced to be inactive almost immediately lose more than 75% of their ability to remove harmful fats from their blood. Humans recorded a 40 percent reduction in insulin's ability to uptake glucose—after only 24 hours of being sedentary.

Let's have a look at some solutions from inactivity researchers and others. Some "get moving" techniques are high tech—and expensive. Others cost little, if anything, and may work just as well. They're all thought provoking.

We'll start with individual examples, and then move on to what researchers are doing for themselves.

Former Secretary of Defense Donald Rumsfeld was a real stand-up guy. There were no chairs in his office. "When he works, he stands. When he reads or writes, he uses a stand-up desk all day," a spokeswoman said. "He's in great shape," she added.

Rumsfeld just turned 80 slim and healthy, so he must still to be standing—and probably doing a lot more. His mind, memory—and wit—are razor sharp. (I saw him on TV yesterday, as I write this.)

Lynn McFarlin, my doctor at the Cooper Clinic, delights in demonstrating his customized desk which at the push of a button becomes a standup work station. He told me that he switches to the stand-up mode in the afternoon when the last patient has left. I didn't ask how much he paid for the desk, but he says it's great for his quirky back, so it must be worth the price. His weight doesn't seem to change from year to year, when I see him.

Some adventurous souls are going further; they're using treadmill desks or work stations that cost as much as $4,000, maybe more. The idea is to slowly walk on the treadmill while working, according to Dr. Levine, who came up with the idea. His says people burn about 100 extra calories every hour while walking slowly—at 1 mile per hour—rather than sitting in a chair.

Dr. Levine uses one himself and knows many others who do. Some have lost up to 40 pounds in a year, he says. He lost 20 pounds.

Some sit on an exercise ball while they work, to use muscles in their back, legs, and abdomen in a way that chairs don't.

Others keep small dumbbells under their desk to use during breaks.

A gym owner told me years ago never to lie down when I could sit up, sit when I could stand, or walk when I could run. Golf was his least favorite game—because the better you get, the fewer strokes you need to win the match. I don't know about the golf analogy, but the general idea has many applications at home and on the job.

Never take the elevator when you can conveniently take the stairs. Stand up when you talk on the telephone. Instead of sending an e-mail, walk down the hall and deliver the message in person when you can.

Park your car within walking distance of your office or work place or on the far side of the department store parking lot.

And, of course, take frequent breaks at home or work; walk

around, stretch, do some push-ups, whatever appeals to you. Roll around on the floor with your kids—or your wife/husband.

Go for a walk when you're trying to solve a problem or have brain lock. You'll be amazed how quickly the answer pops into your head.

Use your imagination. Program movement into your day. You'll feel better, think better, and be more productive. You'll also be leaner and probably live longer.

* * *

We could talk for a very long time about the almost limitless benefits of movement. Instead, let's focus on two major areas of concern—combating creeping obesity and blood sugar swings. (We'll end the chapter with a newly discovered benefit that sounds more like science fiction than science.)

Walking Combats Obesity

Obesity increases the risk of just about everything up to and including death. It typically comes on gradually over many years. A study by researchers at the University of North Carolina found that walking can curb it.

"There is a large body of research on physical activity and weight loss, but little on the amount of exercise needed for long-term weight maintenance," Miriam Nelson, a professor of physical activity and nutrition at Tufts University, wrote in an editorial accompanying the North Carolina study.

The new study addressed that issue.

"This study is the first to demonstrate that walking has an independent protective effect on weight gain," Dr. Nelson observed.

Researchers led by Penny Gordon-Larsen, PhD, followed 4,995 men and women for 15 years to determine whether regular walking is an effective way to counter our tendency to gain weight with age. The results were reported in *The American Journal of Clinical Nutrition* (January 2009).

The participants, from four U.S. cities, ranging in age from 18 to 30, were examined initially and again at 2, 5, 7, 10, and 15 years.

The average weight gain for all subjects was about 2.2 pounds per year—30-plus pounds over 15 years. Two pounds a year doesn't sound like much—but the end result is large.

"We found a substantial association between walking and annualized weight change," the researchers reported. There was a dose effect. Participants who walked the most were most likely to lose or maintain weight: Two hours a week helped keep weight off, but four hours was more effective.

The greatest benefit was seen in women who weighed the most at the beginning of the study and walked the most. For the heaviest 25% of women, those with the highest walking levels were "associated with 17.6 pounds less weight gain over 15 years" compared with women who didn't walk.

The walkers still gained weight, but the yearly gain was 1.17 pounds *less* than the non-walkers.

For the heaviest women, each 30 minutes per day of walking "was associated with an annual reduced weight gain of 1 pound or 15 pounds over 15 years," the researchers wrote.

Men and women in all weight categories who walked were more likely to lose or maintain weight than non-walkers.

"Walking throughout adulthood may attenuate the long-term weight gain that occurs in most adults," Dr. Gordon-Larsen and her colleagues concluded.

This is a big deal. Studies such as this should motivate more people to walk regularly. Walking is a pleasant activity. It gives you energy and makes you feel good. Almost anyone can do it. And it's free.

"If we can increase walking participation by Americans, the evidence is strong that we will improve not only weight control but overall public health," Miriam Nelson concluded at the end of her editorial.

One more important point: Subjects in this study were *not* on a diet or doing other forms of exercise. The reported results were almost surely from walking alone. It's fair to assume that the results would've been better if the subjects had eaten less— but they apparently didn't. Add regular strength training, and results would likely have been better still.

Carol and I have been walking throughout our married life. Walking works!

* * *

Now, let's look at the relationship between physical activity and blood sugar stability.

Another Reason to Keep Moving

We know that inactivity is harmful. It may surprise you to know that we're just beginning to uncover the underlying mechanisms. Why does inactivity make us sick and shorten our lives? How does staying active protect us?

There are reasons why we are slow to unravel the magic of movement and the hazards of inactivity. Studying the harmful effects is hard. Sedentary people may also be obese, eat poorly, or have other health or lifestyle issues that make it almost impossible to determine the role of activity alone.

Scientists from the University of Missouri cleverly removed the uncertainty by persuading healthy young adults to slow down, to stop being so active. They then monitored blood sugar rise and fall, because that is known to be a significant prognosticator. "Spikes and swings in blood sugar after meals have been linked to the development of heart disease and type 2 diabetes," explained John P. Thyfault, an associate professor of nutrition and exercise physiology, who conducted the study along with his graduate student Catherine R. Mikus and others. The results were reported in the February, 2012, *Medicine & Science in Sport & Exercise*. (The study was also chronicled by Gretchen Reynolds in *The New York Times*.)

Thyfault's active young volunteers cut their steps from 10,000 or more a day to less than 5,000 steps. They did it by taking the elevator rather than using the stairs, and driving to work or the corner store rather than walking or biking, and other common energy saving maneuvers. Blood sugar changes were monitored continuously for three days at both levels of activity. Diets were standardized for all subjects; they kept food diaries and ate the same during both study periods.

Ten thousand step days were routine for the participants (average age 29); the average was actually around 13,000 steps during the first monitoring period. The American Heart Association and other groups recommend at least 10,000 steps per day, the equivalent of about five miles of walking. The average American adult takes fewer than 5,000 steps a day—and 79 million of us are currently estimated to be prediabetic.

The study participants cut back to about 4,300 steps on average during the second monitoring period.

During the three days of normal (for them) activity, the volunteers' blood sugar did not spike after they ate; it fluctuated, but not abnormally. It was another story altogether during the three days of reduced activity.

Cutting activity in half for three days wasn't enough to change fitness or body composition, but it did make a considerable difference in blood sugar peaks after meals. Blood sugar peaks increased by about 26 percent compared to when the subjects were exercising and moving more. Moreover, peaks grew higher with each successive day of inactivity. Blood sugar variability after meals increased by as much as twofold.

Think about that. Only three days of reduced activity—on par with the activity level of most Americans—put healthy young adults on track to develop type 2 diabetes and perhaps heart disease. Is it any wonder that one third of Americans are predicted to have type 2 diabetes by the year 2050?

Thyfault assured Gretchen Reynolds that blood sugar control would return to normal once activity resumed. If inactivity continued, however, if it becomes a habit, it would likely become a serious concern. "We hypothesize that, over time, inactivity creates the physiological conditions that produce chronic disease," like type 2 diabetes and heart disease.

Chalk up another rock-solid reason to keep moving. Even a single day of moderate- to vigorous-activity has been shown to improve insulin sensitivity, according to the Thyfault-Mikus team.

Professor Thyfault walks his talk. "When I'm really busy, I make sure to get up and walk around the office or jog in place every hour or so," he told Reynolds. You don't have to get your activity in big doses; your can do it a little at a time, throughout the day. "You don't have to run marathons," Thyfault confirmed. "But the evidence is clear that you do need to move."

* * *

I don't own a pedometer, but Carol has been wearing one for over three years. She has logged an average of 9,800 steps per day over that time. About half is hiking and other forms of exercise; she walked on most days early on, but cut back when she started doing more weight workouts. The balance is made up of daily activities at home, at the office, or being out and about. As Dr. Thyfault suggested, physical activity can come in many forms.

Active living is a mindset. Carol and I enjoy movement; we make it part of our lifestyle. Our favorite movie theater is downtown, a 30-minute drive from our home. We park in a four story parking structure; everyone does, it's the only reliable place to park in that area. What sets us apart is that we always park on the top floor and walk up and down the stairs. The elevator is slow; we never use it. (She beats me up the stairs if I slow down; she always beats me going down.) That's just one example of how we make movement a regular—and fun—part of our life.

Something I've added recently is a little routine I call "Morning Motion." I do it most mornings when I get up, before breakfast, to get my joints moving and my blood flowing.

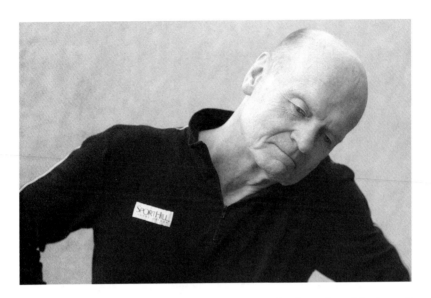

I move my neck as part of my "Morning Motion" routine. Moving all parts of the body is an invigorating way to start the day.

Photo by Laszlo Bencze

I've never timed myself—it varies from day to day—but takes less than 10 minutes. I begin by opening and closing my hands, and then flex and extend my wrists and my elbows, rotate my shoulders and neck, and so on, until I've covered every part of my body. I devote extra time to my lower back, knees, and shoulders. I do overhead movements with a broomstick and an empty bar. I end by doing squats with bodyweight, with the broomstick, and then the bar; 12 or so reps each way, whatever feels right. Morning Motion is a whole body wake-up. I look forward to it.

Like Professor Thyfault, I also get up and move around inside from time to time throughout my day—whenever I need a burst of energy. I also take short walks outside (~10 minutes) at convenient times during the day. Movement makes everything I do go better; it makes me more productive and efficient.

* * *

On days when I don't work out I have always walked. I call it active rest. I believe active rest helps me recover between workouts. Now, research is confirming my belief in spades.

As I said at the beginning of this chapter, movement burns extra calories and speeds recovery—but there's more to it than we could have guessed. That's what the next section is about. It sounds like science fiction—but it's not.

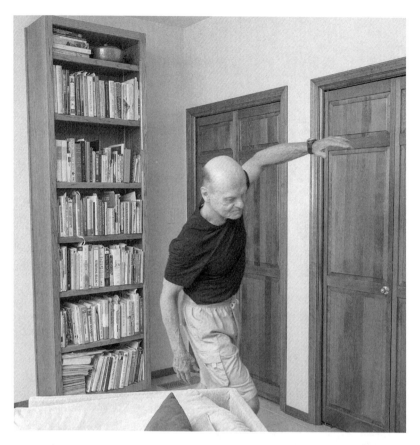

I make a game out of moving around during the day. Here I'm pretending to be an airplane coming in for a landing. *Photo by Laszlo Bencze*

Mother Nature's Recycling and Vitality Mechanism

Scientists believe that we cannibalize our own body parts—in a good way.

It was reported in *The New York Times, Science Daily*, and the *HHMI News*: Mice consume the debris in cells all over their bodies—and exercise stimulates the process.

The Howard Hughes Medical Institute (HHMI) at the University of Texas Southwest Medical Center in Dallas is where much of the research on this process—the technical name is *autophagy*—is being conducted. (The new studies were reported January, 2012, in the journal *Nature*.)

Autophagy means "self-eating." Autophagy is the process

by which cells collect, breakdown, and digest damaged or unneeded parts. It's the body's resourceful way of turning the waste products of cellular function into raw material for new structures or energy. Scientists believe this means of recycling evolved in response to starvation or stress; cells would gather and consume damaged or worn out fragments to keep the rest of the cell alive and healthy. In Petri dishes the rate of autophagy increases when cells are starved or otherwise put under physiological stress. Exercise is a physiological stress. This led researchers to believe that autophagy may explain how exercise fends off metabolic disorders like diabetes and protects against other diseases.

"Autophagy is...known to have several health benefits and those benefits correspond closely to the effects of exercise," said Dr. Beth Levine, professor of internal medicine and microbiology and director of the Center for Autophagy Research at UT Southwestern. "We hypothesized that some of the health benefits of exercise might be explained through autophagy." (Levine is the senior researcher in the new studies and responsible for many of the fundamental discoveries in this area.)

The new research was done in a logical, two-step progression. The first step isolated the effect of exercise on autophagy; and the second step looked at the effects of autophagy. First, they had to determine whether exercise stimulates autophagy, something that had yet to be proven. If so, the next step was to determine the effect of autophagy on fitness and health.

While complex, the research is quite transparent if we take it one step at a time.

As part of the autophagy process a double membrane forms around the unwanted cell fragments as a prelude to breakdown and recycling. The membranes are a marker of autophagy. To test the idea that exercise triggers autophagy, Levine and her colleagues used mice that had been medically treated so that the membranes encasing the debris inside their cells would give off a green glow, signaling that autophagy was taking place. They then placed the mice on treadmills; after 30 minutes of running, the mice had more glowing membranes in cells throughout their bodies. This told the researchers that exercise was sparking autophagy.

"That was a brand new finding," Dr. Levine said. They established—for the first time—that exercise stimulates autophagy. With the exercise connection established, Levine and her colleagues moved on to test the purpose served by autophagy. What does it do? This phase was extended as the effects of autophagy unfolded; one effect opened the door to test another effect.

As noted, previous findings led Dr. Levine to believe that there might be an exercise-autophagy-diabetes connection. The connection was confirmed, but it took several steps.

The Levine team engineered mice that show autophagy under normal circumstances, but lack the ability to ramp up the debris-eating process when stressed. This set the stage for testing the role of autophagy. They then subjected the mutant mice to several phases of testing.

They found that autophagy aids endurance—it allows normal mice to run longer—but it also does more. Without the ability to ramp-up autophagy, the mice were in trouble.

When the researchers placed the autophagy-challenged mice on treadmills, they found that they couldn't run as long as normal mice. A closer look showed that the mice were not metabolizing sugar normally; they weren't burning sugar to fuel their running. As a result, blood sugar levels soared and endurance tanked.

This suggested to the Levine team that the autophagy-deficient mice might also be unable to derive the long-term benefits of exercise. To test this proposition, they fed both mutant and normal mice a high-fat diet for four weeks. *Both mice groups remained sedentary.* Not surprisingly, all of the mice gained weight and developed signs of type 2 diabetes.

They then put the mice (both groups) on a stringent exercise program for eight weeks *while continuing to feed them a high-fat diet.* The normal mice responded, losing weight and pulling back from diabetes. The mutant mice that exercised on the treadmill also lost weight, but did not get the metabolic benefits; their blood sugar remained high.

To get the benefits of exercise, "autophagy really was necessary," Levine happily concluded.

Notably, the Levine team had earlier reported that exercise sparked an increase in autophagy in cells in the liver and pancreas, organs involved in the metabolism of glucose (sugar). This, of course, added another link between exercise, autophagy, and blood sugar regulation.

"Our finding that exercise fails to improve glucose metabolism in autophagy-deficient mice strongly suggests that autophagy is an important mechanism by which exercise protects against diabetes," said Dr. Levine. "It also raises the possibility that activation of autophagy may contribute to other health benefits of exercise, including protection against cancer, neurodegenerative diseases and aging."

Exercise is shaping up to be a miracle elixir for mice and, hopefully, men. Only time—and more research—will tell.

In the meantime, Dr. Levine is taking no chances. She bought a treadmill and resolved to exercise more consistently. "If it's good enough for my mice," she said, "It's good enough for me."

* * *

My take is that autophagy revitalizes the cells in our bodies. Staying active energizes the process.

Dr. Levine's landmark discoveries on exercise and autophagy have me visualizing my cells shedding the flotsam of living on my walks. I listen to the birds sing, and think about my cells becoming more efficient and healthier with each step I take. That's important; the more we understand about the benefits of movement and exercise, the more motivated we are to fill our days with physical activity.

Thank goodness for Beth Levine and other scientists like her. They are showing us the many ways movement and exercise can enhance our lives.

* * *

The couch potato's dream is an exercise pill; pop a pill and grab the remote. Who needs running flats or a barbell? Bye-bye fitness center fees. The pharmaceutical company that develops a pill that mimics the effects of exercise will make Apple and Amazon look like penny stocks.

Arnie Jensen, my original doctor and friend at the Cooper Clinic in Dallas, insisted that we already have an exercise pill. He explained with a twinkle in his eye that it just takes about an hour three times a week to swallow it.

We've discussed the latest findings on exercise and longevity, and how physical activity between workouts keeps our blood circulating and our body purring. Now, let's look at the effect of exercise on specific diseases. The good news keeps coming. It's nothing short of miraculous.

Chapter Eight

Fitness & Health

Miracle of Movement

My mother often protested that I believed exercise was the cure for everything. Well, according to the 2008 book *Move Yourself: The Cooper Clinic Medical Director's Guide to All the Healing Benefits of Exercise (Even a Little!)*, exercise does make everything better. "Our research says that however long you live, every day of your life will be far better if you are involved in physical activity," wrote Drs. Tedd Mitchell and Tim Church, and health writer Martin Zucker. "Statistically you improve the quantity, and in the process you definitely improve the quality."

The authors tell us that the "first dramatic scientific breakthrough" came in 1953 when Jeremy Morris, a British researcher, found that conductors who constantly walk up and down collecting tickets on London's famous double-decker buses enjoyed better health and had fewer heart attacks than drivers who sat immobile for 90% of their shift. Morris reinforced his findings with another study showing that postmen who walk or cycle carrying the mail had fewer heart attacks than sedentary telephone operators and clerks.

The evidence since then on the benefits of exercise has continued to mount exponentially. Inactivity has been elevated to major status as a risk factor. Based on evidence from the Cooper Clinic and elsewhere, sedentary living is now given the same status as smoking, high blood pressure, high cholesterol, and obesity as a predictor of health and longevity.

We already know that exercise helps control body fat, cholesterol levels, and blood pressure, and that it improves fitness. Let's look at some of the lesser known benefits. Some of them are surprising and all of them are encouraging to those of us who want to do everything we reasonably can to live healthy longer.

Mitchell and Church say there is an exciting new focus in the control of diabetes—on muscle. We now have a greater appreciation for the fact that muscles both consume and store blood sugar. Skeletal muscles, the muscles that move the body, are the body's biggest consumer of blood sugar. "When you aren't active, your muscles don't use or store glucose in a normal, efficient way," the doctors explained. "When the muscle cells don't open up for sugar intake, as happens in the prediabetic state of insulin resistance, the sugar builds up in the blood." Muscles burn blood sugar during exercise—and exercise makes muscles more receptive to the storage of sugar for future use, when you exercise again.

"The impact of physical activity on blood sugar is spectacular," the doctors wrote. Blood sugar drops almost immediately. "If you are physically active today, your body will process glucose better the rest of the day, and tomorrow, and even the day after," the doctors report. "You can practically argue that nothing in the body responds so positively and so quickly to physical activity as blood sugar."

The first hard evidence that physical activity is protective against cancer came in 1922, when two independent studies showed that men from Australia, England, and the United States who did "hard muscular work" had lower rates of cancer than those doing less physically demanding jobs. The medical community didn't pay much attention at the time, according to Mitchell and Church, and the idea dropped from sight until recent years, when evidence again began to accumulate.

In 1989, a major study from the Cooper Clinic, based on more than 13,000 patients followed for eight years, showed a "powerful link" between fitness level and death rates from all illnesses, including cancer. In 1996, another study by a Cooper Clinic researcher involving 25,000 patients "showed that physically active men had a much lower risk of dying from cancer than nonactive men." The fittest men (top 20%) had a cancer death rate 81 percent lower than the least fit 20%.

Precisely how exercise protects against cancer is unclear, but Mitchell and Church said scientists believe that exercise stimulates the body's ability to fight off cancer in various ways.

"Every day we have cells that turn cancerous," the doctors related. "The body needs to eliminate them." A sedentary body "works sluggishly," and simply doesn't do the job as well as a fit body. Exercise bolsters the ability of our immune system "to clean house."

The evidence of the protective benefits of exercise is especially strong for some types of cancer. Dr. I-Min Lee, a member for the Cooper Clinic Scientific Advisory Board and an assistant professor of medicine at Harvard, is an expert on the role of exercise in the prevention of cancer. Lee said the association between physical activity and prevention is strongest for colon cancer, lung cancer, ovarian cancer, and breast cancer.

Exercise also wards off osteoporosis and depression. You probably knew that. But did you know that it also gives you more energy, and helps you sleep better?

It might seem counterintuitive that exercise, which tires you out, also makes you more energetic—but it's true. It's a simple matter of use it or lose it. "Our bodies are made to be used," the doctors write. Use it more and it gives you more.

Mitchell and Church did a quality-of-life survey for their book involving 10,000 patients. Among the many things they found is that "physical activity is a great energy booster." Twenty six percent of patients with low fitness reported unexplained fatigue, compared to 16 percent for moderately fit patients—and only 11 percent for high-fit patients.

"Sedentary living robs you of energy," the doctors write. "Physical activity brings it back and reduces fatigue."

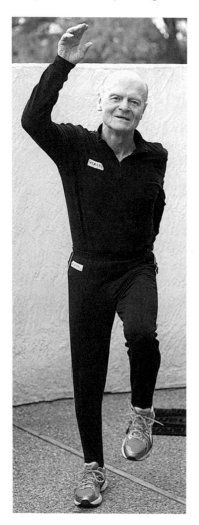 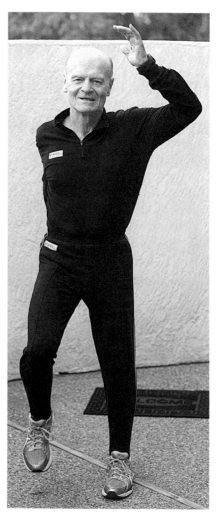

Our bodies are made to move. Use it more and it gives you more

Photos by Laszlo Bencze

"Physical activity makes all the body's systems operate better, from top to bottom," the doctors stated. "As a by-product, your body generates more energy."

That's really what exercise is about, isn't it? Tire the body, let it rest, and you'll tire less easily the next time. Stress, rest, and improve.

The flip side is that you'll also sleep more soundly at night if you exercise and tire yourself out during the day.

"Keep in mind that nature is based on cycles of rest and activity," the doctors counseled. "If you don't get enough of one, the other is affected."

"Sleep has a great deal to do with energy," they explain. If you exercise during the day, "instead of waking up with the battery 75 percent or less charged, you wake up fully charged." Drain your battery during the day and "fall asleep faster and experience more restful and restorative sleep."

This advice works best, Mitchell and Church tell their patients, if exercise and sleep are scheduled properly. They emphasize two important don'ts.

1. Don't sacrifice sleep to exercise early in the morning. Adjust your day to fit in exercise. If you don't get enough sleep, it makes you less productive in everything you do, including exercise. What's more, the doctors say sleep deprivation makes you produce less leptin, the satiety hormone, causing you to eat more and gain weight. Make a firm appointment with yourself to exercise during the day, and keep it.

2. Don't exercise shortly before going to bed. That makes it harder to fall asleep. "You put your body into a physiologically excited state," the doctors explain, "that makes it harder to settle down."

* * *

Drs. Mitchell and Church explained generally how exercise combats cancer. Some other researchers, from Finland, Sweden, and elsewhere, are filling in the details. Interestingly, different forms of exercise seem to have different benefits.

Strength and Fitness Fight Cancer Independently

One study deals with the relationship between intensity and cancer mortality. Another evaluates the benefits of weight training following treatment for breast cancer. Finally, we have a comprehensive study which examines muscular strength, body fat, and aerobic fitness as cancer predictors.

We'll look at the studies separately, and then together.

The study from Finland, first published in the *British Journal of Sports Medicine* on July 28, 2009, found that at least 30 minutes a day of moderate to high intensity physical activity cut cancer deaths in half.

Some have proposed that the volume of physical activity—burning 1,000 calories a week, for example—is as or more important than the type, frequency, or intensity of the activity. The aim of the Finish study was to assess the role of intensity in the reduction of cancer mortality. Is picking berries or fishing as effective as running, skiing, or lifting weights?

Exercise intensity was measured in metabolic equivalents of oxygen consumption (METs). (One MET is defined as the oxygen uptake when a person is at rest.) For example, the average oxygen uptake of running was 10.1 METs, biking to work was 5.8 METs, picking berries was 3.6 METs, and fishing was 2.4 METs.

Here's what they found.

Men with leisure-time physical activity averaging more than 5.2 METs (highest quartile) were found to have half the risk of dying from cancer compared to men with an average intensity level of 3.7 METs (lowest quartile).

The fitness of the participants was also measured. "An increase of 1 MET of physical fitness amounted to a 12% reduced risk in cancer death," the researchers reported.

So, intensity level does make a difference.

"Intensity should be at least moderate so that the beneficial effect of physical activity for reducing overall cancer mortality can be achieved," the researchers wrote. "Anything above an average of 4 MET can be considered moderate-intensity exercise," said Sudhir Kurl, MD, the lead researcher.

Asked if he practices what he preaches, Dr. Kurl replied: "Of course!" He jogs 3 times a week and works out in the gym twice a week. (I interpret that to mean that he lifts weights twice a week.)

That brings us to weight training for breast-cancer survivors.

"For many years; we told [breast-cancer survivors] not to lift anything heavier than a handbag," said Anna Schwartz, an affiliate professor of nursing. "This is the first really well-designed study that demonstrates that women can do a lot more than we thought."

The impediment is lymphedema, one of the most troubling complications that can develop after treatment for breast cancer. Lymphedema is swelling caused by build up of lymph fluid after the patient's lymph nodes are removed or interrupted during surgery or radiation. The swelling causes discomfort and pain in the arms and hands.

Women are advised to ask for help with shopping bags, avoid picking up children, and to stick with milder forms of exercise, such as walking, swimming, and light aerobics. Weight lifting is a definite "no-no."

A new study by Kathryn H. Schmitz, PhD, MPH, University of Pennsylvania School of Medicine, and colleagues, published August 13, 2009, in the *New England Journal of Medicine*, showed that the dangers of resistance training may have been overblown—that strength training may actually be a substantial help to women struggling with lymphedema.

The study randomly assigned 141 middle-aged breast-cancer survivors with stable lymphedema to a twice weekly 90-minute progressive weight lifting program or a control group that did no lifting.

The lifting started with "little-to-no resistance." As long as no signs of flare-up were noted, resistance was progressively increased by "the smallest possible increments." No upper limits were placed on the weight to which women could progress in any exercise. In short, they tried hard to do no harm.

Importantly, there were "no serious adverse events related to the intervention."

At the end of the study the women who lifted were substantially stronger than the controls. "Slowly progressive weight lifting had no significant effect on limb swelling and resulted in a decreased incidence of exacerbation of lymphedema, reduced symptoms, and increased strength," the report concluded.

Lead author Kathryn Schmitz, an exercise physiologist, is optimistic that the study will change doctors' advice on weight training to lymphedema-sufferers. "Hopefully this will be the last nail in the coffin for that kind of misguided advice," she told reporters.

The third and last study looks at muscular strength, fatness, and cardiovascular fitness as cancer predictors. Led by Jonatan R. Ruiz of the Department of Biosciences and Nutrition at the Karolinska Institute in Hudding, Sweden, the study is reported in *Cancer Epidemiology, Biomarkers & Prevention* (May 2009).

The study involved 8,677 men (age 20 to 80) who received

comprehensive medical exams, including muscular strength and aerobic fitness testing at the Cooper Clinic. Body composition was also measured as part of the exam. During an average follow-up period of 18.9 years, 503 of the men died, 199 from cancer and 145 from cardiovascular disease.

There were three main findings.

First, muscular strength was significantly and inversely associated with cancer mortality; men in the moderate and high strength category had about 37% fewer cancer deaths than those in the lowest strength category. This association remained after adjustment for overall and waistline fatness, and for cardiovascular fitness.

Secondly, percent body fat was positively associated with rates of cancer mortality; higher body fat was associated with higher rates of cancer deaths. This association, however, did not persist after adjustment for muscular strength or cardiovascular fitness. In other words, higher strength and fitness appear to substantially override higher body fat.

Third, a combination of muscular strength and fatness is powerfully associated with cancer death; men in the *lowest* third for muscular strength with high levels of fatness have a 40% to 50% higher rate of cancer death than obese men with at least moderate (middle third) muscular strength. In short, a moderate level of muscular strength counts for a lot if you are overweight.

"Taken together, these findings indicate that having at least moderate age-adjusted levels of muscular strength may counteract the deleterious consequences attributed to adiposity," the report stated. "Efforts should then focus not only on reducing levels of adiposity *but also on increasing the muscular strength level.*" (Emphasis mine)

Now we shift focus to cardiovascular fitness. Listen to what Ruiz and his colleagues say about the importance of aerobic fitness: "Higher levels of cardiorespiratory fitness are strongly associated with lower risk of cancer mortality in men and women, young or older people, and in diabetic or nondiabetic persons, independently of their weight status and tobacco use." Clearly, aerobic fitness has a powerful effect on cancer risk.

Men who were strong but *unfit* were at appreciably higher risk than men who were strong and *fit*.

Interestingly, the study found that muscular strength and cardiorespiratory fitness were only "moderately correlated." This suggests that the associations between the two forms of fitness and cancer risk involve "different mechanisms." Both strength and aerobic fitness appear to have profound *and independent* effects on cancer risk. A combination of the two forms of fitness, working together, would appear to be most protective.

Age-adjusted death rate in men with high levels of *both muscular strength and cardiovascular fitness* was 60% lower than the death rate in unfit men with the lowest level of muscular strength. Unquestionably, it pays to be both fit and strong.

Leanness, of course, remains important. "Maintaining a healthy weight should continue to be a cornerstone in the prevention of chronic disease and premature death," Ruiz and his colleagues emphasized.

* * *

The simple regimen of Sudhir Kurl, MD, the lead researcher in the study from Finland, embodies the new science-based prescription for fitness and health. He jogs and he lifts.

Yes, I know; that's the old formula. The difference is that we now have a much better understanding of why it works so well.

* * *

Let's shift gears and talk about the role of exercise in maintaining mental health.

The Awesome Power of Exercise— Help for Schizophrenics

A study reported in the February 2010 issue of *Archives of General Psychiatry* found that aerobic exercise can significantly increase hippocampal volume in the brains of patients with schizophrenia—and in healthy controls. That's good news for everyone.

The hippocampus plays a major part in brain function. Damage to that region of the brain is known to cause memory problems and disorientation.

Schizophrenia is a mysterious disease characterized by gross distortion of reality. While the causes are not well understood, numerous abnormalities of brain structures have been reported. Many researchers have found reduced hippocampus size in schizophrenic subjects.

The authors observed that "exercise is a stimulus to hippocampal plasticity" in healthy individuals. Connecting the dots, they decided to use aerobic exercise to "probe into the capacity of the hippocampus for plasticity in schizophrenia." Happily, they found that plasticity is present. (Brain plasticity means the ability to grow or change.)

"The therapeutic options for schizophrenia are not really good, and we're convinced that schizophrenia is a brain disease [characterized by] a lack of neuroplasticity," said lead researcher Frank-Gerald Pajonk, MD, Department of Psychiatry and Psychotherapy, The Saarland University Hospital, Homburg, Germany. "So we wanted to look at solutions that could possibly improve this deficit."

"These results indicate that in [these patients], hippocampal volume is plastic in response to aerobic exercise," wrote Dr. Pajonk and his colleagues.

"To our knowledge, this is the first time that it has been shown that the hippocampus is growing in patients with schizophrenia," Dr. Pajonk told *Medscape Psychiatry*.

"As the hippocampus is one of the core structures in schizophrenia, we were thinking that if there was an increase in volume, it could give some improvement in cognition," Pajonk added. "And that's what we found."

The details are intriguing and encouraging—for all of us.

The study included 16 adult males with chronic schizophrenia and eight matched healthy controls. Those with schizophrenia were randomly assigned to an exercise program consisting of 30 minutes of supervised cycling three times a week for three months, or to play tabletop football for the same amount of time. Half of the patients cycled and the other half played tabletop football. All eight healthy controls took part in the cycling program.

All participants underwent magnetic resonance imaging (MRI) of the hippocampus, as well as neuropsychological and clinical testing. In addition, all subjects were tested for aerobic fitness.

Notably, hippocampal volume was 4% smaller in the schizophrenic patients before exercise training.

Hippocampal volume increased in all participants who cycled, by 12% in those with schizophrenia and 16% in the healthy controls; there was no change in those who played tabletop football. Significantly, changes in hippocampal volume were correlated with improvement in aerobic fitness.

"To provide a context," the authors wrote, "the magnitude of these changes in volume was similar to that observed for other [deep brain] structures when patients were switched from typical to atypical antipsychotic drug therapy." Exercise had effects similar to potent drugs, without the possible side effects.

Short-term memory scores also improved. The patients in the schizophrenia exercise group showed a 34% improvement in short-term memory after the exercise program, while schizophrenia patients who did not exercise scored 6% lower. Tellingly, for the combined exercise and non-exercise schizophrenia group, changes in short-term memory were correlated with change in hippocampal volume. Increase in volume went hand in hand with improved memory.

In the schizophrenia exercise group—but not in the healthy controls—change in hippocampal volume was associated with a 35% increase in the N-acetylaspartate, "a marker of neuronal [brain cell] integrity." The authors are not sure what this means, but it could suggest that the brains cells of the schizophrenia patients were more in need of repair or renewal.

Finally, the severity of total symptoms of schizophrenia improved somewhat in the exercise group—9% lower—and worsened in the non-exercise group—13% higher.

Impressive—and there's more.

"Although I can't prove it right now, I'm positive that exercise is doing good in the treatment of schizophrenia," Dr. Pajonk opined enthusiastically. "Many of the schizophrenia patients from the [cycling] groups were able to go on and develop a life of their own, moving to a new apartment, taking up a job again, etc. It's a bit early and we just had a small sample size, but with this small number of patients, we were really surprised and amazed at what has happened to them."

Christopher A. Ross, MD, PhD, director of the Division of Neurobiology and professor of psychiatry at Johns Hopkins School of Medicine, who did not take part, called the study "interesting" with implications beyond schizophrenia. "In a sense, this was more a study about the brain and plasticity than schizophrenia per se," he told *Medscape Psychiatry*. "The good news is that the brain is much more plastic than we had previously appreciated," he continued. "Just something like exercising may alter a significant feature of brain structure."

* * *

This study shows the awesome power of exercise to improve brain function.

We must not forget, however, that "use it or lose it" still applies. Dr. Pajonk clearly suggests that many of the patients who exercised used their new and improved brain volume to make a better life for themselves.

Exercise creates an environment conducive to change, but you must give your brain a reason to change, a new challenge.

The schizophrenia patients responded to their challenge in ways they were unable to without exercise. The rest of us need to do the same. We must exercise our body and challenge our brain.

* * *

I prefer intervals over steady state aerobics. Intervals are more efficient and more interesting. And the advantages don't stop there. A new study from Brazil highlights an important health advantage of stop and go exercise.

Interval Training Reduces Arterial Stiffness

It seems logical that interval training would be more effective than steady-state exercise in improving blood vessel flexibility. And that's what a new study performed by researchers at the University of Sao Paulo found. Dr. Guilherme Veiga Guimaraes and his colleagues reported their findings in the April 9, 2010, online edition of *Hypertension Research.*

Exercise has been shown to lower blood pressure and reduce arterial stiffness, but it has not been established which type of exercise does this best. Steady-state continuous exercise is the most common form of exercise, and is typically recommended for people with high blood pressure.

"Interval training promotes greater gradients of shear stress because patients fluctuate between high and low intensities," Dr. Guimaraes and his colleagues wrote in introducing their study. "We have recently shown that interval exercise acutely decreases blood pressure in hypertensive patients," they added. "We therefore hypothesized that interval exercise has a better effect on arterial stiffness and blood pressure control than continuous exercise does on hypertensive subjects."

The aim of the study was to test that hypothesis. Here's how they went about it and what they found.

Sixty-five sedentary patients with controlled hypertension were randomly assigned to three different regimens for 16 weeks: continuous exercise (26), intervals (26), or a sedentary control routine (13).

Continuous exercise was 40 minutes at 60% of reserve heart rate. (Reserve heart rate is the difference between peak and resting heart rate.) Interval exercise was 40 minutes with intensity alternating between 50% (two minutes) and 80% (one minute). Average heart rate was 60% under both routines. The only difference was the up-and-down intensity in the interval group.

At the end of the 16-week study, training method (continuous or interval) made no significant difference in blood pressure; both forms of exercise reduced blood pressure. There was, however, a distinction in the effect on arterial stiffness.

Blood pressure declined most in subjects with higher readings at the beginning of the study. Training protocol, continuous or interval, made no difference.

Training protocol did, however, make a major difference in arterial stiffness as shown by changes in blood flow speed. Flexibility increases the time it takes blood to flow from one point to another.

Sixteen weeks of interval training significantly decreased— speeded up—the time for pulse waves to travel from the neck to the groin. (Transit time also improved after 16 weeks of continuous training, but the change was not statistically significant.) Guimaraes and his colleagues concluded: "Continuous and interval exercise training were beneficial for blood pressure control, but only interval training reduced arterial stiffness."

The researchers gave their finding more punch by explaining that aging typically leads to a progressive increase in arterial stiffness, especially in larger arteries. Not surprisingly, increase in stiffness is more pronounced in those with high blood pressure.

"Aerobic exercise training seems to attenuate arterial stiffness in healthy subjects, but the results in hypertensive patients are controversial," the researchers related. That, of course, makes their finding regarding the effect of interval training on stiffness in hypertensive patients more meaningful.

"Arterial stiffness has been shown to be an independent predictor of cardiovascular and all-cause mortality in hypertensive patients," the researchers observed. "Sedentary lifestyle and anti-hypertensive treatment resulted in an increase [slowing] of 0.8ms [millisecond] of pulse wave velocity in 6 years," they added.

"*Our study shows that only 16 weeks of interval training caused a drop in* pulse wave velocity *of 0.41ms in a similar population.*" (Emphasis mine)

In other words, interval training halved 6 years of arterial stiffening in only 16 weeks!

The researchers also provided a similar statistic for blood pressure: "It has been documented that a reduction of only 2mmHg in systolic blood pressure [the top number] decreases mortality from cerebral accidents by 10% and cardiovascular disease by 7%."

In their study, the drop in systolic pressure was 7mmHg and 6mmHg for continuous and interval training, respectively.

To recap briefly, continuous and interval training reduced blood pressure about the same, but only intervals significantly improved arterial stiffness. Add that intervals improve fitness in less time and are more appealing, and it's a slam dunk for intervals.

*　*　*

I always strive to improve in one way or another. That's what keeps me training. Making progress toward a meaningful goal keeps me motivated. It turns out that it also keeps me exceptionally healthy.

Physical Activity Matters, Fitness Matters More

We have been constantly told to keep moving, but rarely are we urged to move fast and become more fit. Until Now.

In 1989, a well-publicized study from the Cooper Institute in Dallas reported that the greatest benefits come when we move from "unfit" (the bottom 20 %) to the medium-fitness group (the next 40%). Those in the high-fitness group were found to be only slightly better off than those in the medium-fitness groups. In other words, high-fitness mattered, but not much.

Exercise is often presented as a "no sweat" proposition. A little effort is said to produce large benefits. That's a good thing to the extent it gets people off the couch, but it's only the beginning.

The big picture is starting to come into focus. We are learning that the greatest benefits come from high levels of fitness. We applaud those who are physically active, but they should know that substantially greater benefits are there for the taking. Effort makes a difference. Serious training produces serious rewards.

It's time to stop thinking about the (almost) free lunch, and start thinking about fitness.

We have two recent studies: the first one spotlights pace and the second fitness level.

Now that most of us are living past 70, the goal has shifted to achieving that age in exceptional health.

Dr. Qi Sun and a team of researchers from Harvard and England examined data from 13,535 nurses over 15 years looking for successful survivors—defined as survival to 70 or older with no chronic diseases, impairment in cognitive function, or physical disability. Fewer than 11% (1456) cleared the hurdle. Nurses who were physically active at midlife (age 60 here) were found to have better odds of exceptional health at age 70.

But there's more. Women with a moderate walking pace had a 90% increase in the odds of successful aging. A "brisk" or "very brisk" pace, however, increased odds 2.68-fold. (*Archives of Internal Medicine*, January 25, 2010).

In 1986, the researchers started collecting detailed information on physical activity. They inquired about the average time in the past year spent on physical activities—walking, biking, hiking, running, tennis, rowing, dancing and so on. For walkers, they also inquired about usual pace—casual, normal, brisk, and very brisk.

They divided the nurses into categories, based on total physical activity and walking pace. All information was analyzed in relation to successful aging. As noted, physical activity level (amount) and walking pace proved to be good predictors of whether participants were among the 12,079 "Usual Survivors" or the 1,456 "Successful Survivors."

Again, walking pace was the best predictor of successful aging. Odds ratios for casual (<2.0 mph), normal (2.0-2.9 mph), brisk (3.0-3.9 mph), and very brisk (4.0+ mph) were 1, 1.90, and 2.68 (brisk/very brisk), respectively.

Physical activity is a good prognosticator of health status, but pace or intensity provides far better odds on successful aging.

The other study, published online June 1, 2010, in *Hypertension*, draws a bright line between activity and fitness.

Lead author Mercedes R. Carnethon, MD, (Feinberg School on Medicine, Northwestern University) and a diverse team from the U.S. and Norway tested whether physical activity and fitness are independent factors in the incidence of hypertension. The study is one of the first to distinguish physical activity and fitness. That's important, because one is a behavior and the other a physiological measure.

They found that high activity was significantly associated with healthy (non-hypertensive) blood-pressure—but only when fitness levels were highest.

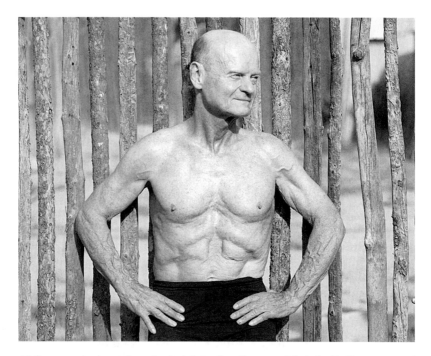

At the conclusion of my last visit to the Cooper Clinic in Dallas, several weeks after this photo was taken, my doctor, Lynn McFarlin, laughed and said, "I can't find anything wrong with you." Effort makes a difference. Serious training produces serious rewards.

Photo by Laszlo Bencze

Dr. Carnethon explained the importance of this finding to *HeartWire* (June 8, 2010): "We know that activity is the principle behavioral determinant of fitness, and we know that being more physically active can improve one's fitness. But the activity needs to be moderate to vigorous to adequately improve fitness [and] see greater health benefits....We are showing this, for the first time, with objective data."

As we said earlier, it takes effort to produce real benefits.

Let's see what they did and what they found.

Carnethon's team analyzed data from 4618 men and women who were initially tested at ages 18 to 30 years in 1985-86 and re-tested 2, 5, 7, 10, 15, and 20 years later. Fitness was measured using a maximum exertion treadmill test, and physical activity was self-reported. The investigation was restricted to initial measures of activity and fitness, while blood pressure was reviewed during the 20-year follow-up period.

While acknowledging that using activity and fitness measures in young adulthood only may be considered a limitation, Carnethon explained that physical activity patterns tend to track over time. Moreover, she emphasizes that their study shows the importance of adopting an active lifestyle early on.

For men and women, those high in fitness had a low incidence of hypertension. By contrast, patterns of association between activity and incidents of hypertension were less pronounced.

A previous analysis of the same information showed that young adults who were the most active were less likely to develop high blood pressure. The current study went beyond the previous analysis to take into account fitness. That's when the benefits of physical activity came into question.

Look carefully at what they found: "There was no evidence of statistical interaction between activity and fitness in association with the development of hypertension. When both were included in the same model, fitness remained significant and independently associated with a lower likelihood of developing hypertension, *whereas activity attenuated to nonsignificance.*" (Emphasis mine)

"Fitness was significantly and inversely associated with the development of hypertension within each [category] of physical activity...Activity was only significantly inversely associated with the development of hypertension *in the highest category of fitness.*" (Emphasis mine)

Physical activity and fitness are independent factors. Activity helps to ward off hypertension—only if fitness level is high. If you are fit, activity level can be low, moderate, or high. Statistically speaking, it doesn't matter.

Dr. Carnethon and her team say their analysis suggests that a third of hypertension cases (34%) could be prevented if participants had moved into a higher fitness category, low to moderate or moderate to high.

* * *

These remarkable studies lend credibility to short, hard, and infrequent aerobic training. That's the formula I follow—mostly in the form of intervals—and my resting heart rate and blood pressure are proof of the pudding. You can train hard or you can train long; it's very difficult to do both. The advantage of interval training is that it allows you to train hard longer.

* * *

Alright, so exercise can help with some physical challenges such as hypertension, diabetes, and cancer, but aren't we at the mercy of our genes? The next section helps to answer that question, and many others. What it shows is that we have the power—largely untapped power—to improve our own health. The opportunity for improvement is stunning

Change Your Lifestyle, Change Your Life

Scientists have known for sometime that a single fat and obesity gene (abbreviated FTO) predisposes people to obesity. In the last three years, however, more DNA variants have been linked to obesity. "The more [gene] variants you carry, the more likely you are to be obese," said Ruth J. F. Loos, program leader at Cambridge University's Medical Research Council Epidemiology Unit.

Loos is the senior author of a powerful study (*PLoS Medicine*, August 31, 2010) to determine the extent to which genetic susceptibility may be overcome by physical activity.

Loos and her team examined the effect of 12 genes associated with a high risk of obesity; the study included 20,430 people. They calculated a genetic predisposition score for each participant ranging from 0 to 24, representing the number of obesity-related genes inherited. Most of the scores were between 10 and 13. They also queried the subjects about their level of physical activity.

They determined that each genetic variant carried a 16 percent increased risk of obesity. For participants who were physically active at least one hour a day, however, the risk was only 10 percent per variant. That's a reduction of 37.5 percent.

In terms of actual weight gain, that translated to 1.3 pounds for each variant in inactive subjects. In people who exercised, the weight gain was only 0.8 pounds, a difference of about 39 percent.

That's big. It means we can do something about genetic predisposition. It's not destiny. It's a tendency that can be overcome or mitigated by lifestyle change. Walking regularly would make a huge difference in the lives of the roughly 225 million sedentary adults. Walking briskly or uphill a couple of times a week and lifting weights 30 minutes twice a week would be even better.

A combination of diet *and* exercise would, no doubt, increase the lifestyle advantage.

What about an ailing heart?

We have long known that exercise reduces the risk of heart

disease. We now have substantial evidence that it can also *reverse* the damage of heart disease. (European Society of Cardiology Congress, Stockholm, Sweden, August 30, 2010)

Dr. Brage Amundsen (Norwegian University of Science and Technology) told the Cardiology Congress what his group is learning about the use of exercise to improve peak oxygen consumption in heart-failure patients.

They compared interval training and continuous exercise in 200 patients.

Preliminary results showed that interval training improved peak oxygen consumption by a much larger margin than continuous training. Specifically, "the interval-training group exhibited...left ventricular remodeling...and improved left ventricular ejection fraction." In plain language, their heart muscle grew stronger and pumped oxygenated blood to their body more forcefully. (There were more signs of improvement, but that's the easiest to understand.)

"It's not that hard and anybody can do it," Dr. Amundsen told the conference. The interval protocol was 4-minutes of brisk walking on a treadmill, with 3-minutes of active rest. The work intervals were at 90% to 95% of peak heart rate and rest periods were at 50-70%. They did four reps for a total of 28 minutes. The continuous-training group walked at 70-75% of heart rate peak for 47 minutes.

Again, interval training produced substantially better results that steady state exercise.

What about the role of strength training?

In a separate presentation, Dr. Francois Carre (Hospital Pontchaillou, Rennes, France) described research showing that cardiovascular-disease patients benefit from strengthening large muscles. (Strong muscles help the heart pump blood throughout the body.) Dr. Carre told the gathering that "well-done" resistance training should be encouraged, that the benefits far outweigh the risks. "The physician must...give a good education to the patients," he explained.

Finally—and perhaps most telling—Dr. Rainer Hambrecht (Herzzentrum Bremen, Germany) told the conference that "only exercise improves [arterial] function and slows the progression of [heart] disease... [Standard patient care] is only a local palliative therapy, while *exercise training has an impact on the underlying disease in the entire coronary tree*," Hambrecht said. (Emphasis mine)

And what about the mind? Is dementia inevitable as we age?

A new analysis of data collected in the renowned Framingham Study indicates that moderate to heavy physical activity reduces the risk of dementia by 45 percent.

"A reduced risk of dementia may be one of the additional health benefits that can be derived from maintaining at least moderate physical activity," lead author Zaldy Tan, MD, MPH, Harvard Medical School, told the International Conference on Alzheimer's Disease 2010 in Honolulu, Hawaii.

"Interestingly, while there are many potentially modifiable risk factors that have been linked with Alzheimer's disease and dementia, physical activity seems to be one that is fairly consistent in being shown to be related to the risk of dementia," Tan said.

A recent review showed that 20 of 24 population-based studies showed a link between physical activity and risk of cognitive decline, Tan added.

"I'm perfectly comfortable with [exercise] being one of our primary recommendations," William Thies, PhD, chief medical and scientific officer of the National Alzheimer's Association, said. The strength of Dr. Tan's paper is that "it comes from a really big, really good, historically dependable study."

Exercise is the nearest thing we have to a sure-fire answer to dementia and AD.

What's more, exercise works at any age.

It's never too late to receive a survival benefit from physical activity, Dr. Peter Kokkinos (Georgetown School of Medicine, Washington DC) told *HeartWire*.

His team tested 5314 males—aged 65 to 92 years—on a treadmill for peak exercise capacity in METs or metabolic equivalents. (Again, one MET is the oxygen uptake at rest.) "Most health benefits are evident at fitness levels of greater than 5 METs," Kokkinos explained.

The study found that each MET increase in exercise capacity carries with it a 12% reduction in the risk of death. Those able to achieve a MET level over 5 had a 38% lower risk of death. The fittest, those with a capacity over 9 METs, had a 61% lower mortality risk.

Kokkinos said there was no difference in the effect of exercise capacity on mortality in older patients; 70-year-olds benefited the same as younger patients. No matter what the age, unfit individuals who improved their exercise capacity to above 5 METs had a 38% lower risk of death.

Again, it's not that hard. Kokkinos stressed that 20 to 40 minutes of brisk daily exercise will move capacity over 5 METs. One patient, a 90-year-old man, returned for follow-up with an exercise capacity of 12 METs, all from daily walking, Kokkinos related.

Fortunately, you don't need a human performance laboratory to gauge your future prospects. Your capacity to do everyday tasks is a strong indicator of vitality—and for some a wake-up call.

British researchers did a systematic review of studies examining the relationship between ability to do physical tasks of everyday living—grip strength, walking speed, chair rising, and standing balance times—and mortality. Their results are reported in the September 9, 2010, *British Medical Journal.*

In every measure, those who performed less well were found to be at a higher risk of all cause mortality. For example, comparing the weakest with the strongest quarter in grip strength (14 studies, 53,475 participants) the risk was 67% higher. For walking speed (5 studies, 14,692 participants) the margin was 187%. For chair-rise time it was 96%.

Standing balance has not been measured and categorized like the other tasks, but all five studies found evidence that poor performance in standing balance tests was associated with higher mortality rates.

Importantly, all of these tasks improve with practice. A well-known study at Tufts University found that wheel-chair bound oldsters, some in their 90s, became mobile again after a short period of strength training.

If you or someone you love is falling behind, do something about it. Fight back. Help yourself. Change your destiny. You have the power.

* * *

What should we eat to stay strong and healthy? As in the case of exercise, we have many healthy choices. The basic dietary guidelines —far fewer than many would have us believe—allow enough flexibility to satisfy almost any palate. The next chapter is about choosing wisely. I'll tell you about my favorite eating pattern and help you find yours.

Chapter Nine

Healthy Eating

U.S. News & World Report Ranks Diets

Many diets are good according to a comprehensive survey by *U.S. News & World Report*. Some diets are better than others for specific purposes, but there are many healthy diets. In their second annual survey, *U.S. News* ranked 25 (up from 20 in 2011) well-known eating plans—for nutrition and safety, short and long term weight loss, heart health, diabetes, and ease of compliance.

Scores were based on reviews by 22 experts in diet and nutrition. The "Best Diets Overall" category combined the ratings in all categories. The magazine also asked readers whether the diets would work for them. (Readers and experts didn't always agree.) The bottom line is that there is no one best diet; there are many that are good. You are most likely to stick with the dietary pattern that you believe in and enjoy.

The Mediterranean Diet (Med Diet), ranked third overall, is my favorite. I'll explain why as we go along. We'll end this section with two new peer-reviewed studies that drive home the benefits of the Mediterranean Diet. An important consideration is the inclusion of fish; we'll talk about that too.

The Med Diet may not work for you; if that's the case, it's for you to decide which diet would suit you. It's an undertaking with the potential to pay dividends for the rest of your life. Thinking carefully—and knowledgably—about what you eat can help you avoid wrong turns you would deeply regret.

While the primary focus of the *U.S. News* ranking is on food, almost all of the diet plans recommend exercise; some give it serious attention and others only lip service. That's an important clue. Any diet plan that down-plays exercise is subject to serious challenge; it may be long on hype and short on sustainable results. Diet and exercise are a winning combination.

Nutritional completeness is another key factor. *U.S. News* looked to the federal government's Dietary Guidelines for Americans 2010 as the benchmark for its "healthy eating" rating. (Keep in mind that government guidelines are based on consensus and not always current on the latest findings.) Most diets passed muster in this category, but a few were taken to task; two or three in particular that I'll tell you about.

Any diet that short-changes fruits, vegetables, or whole grains is suspect. These are the foods that give us the vitamins, minerals, and fiber we need to be healthy—without over-shooting our calorie needs. Protein is another essential nutrient, but most diet plans provide more than enough. Few Americans are deficient in protein; the problem is usually the saturated fat and salt that comes along with it. Finally, good fat is an important dietary component, one which is often overlooked or misunderstood.

We'll talk about some of the top ranked diets, and then a few that didn't fare so well.

The top five "Best Diets Overall" have much in common; the difference is mainly one of emphasis. Four of the five are balanced diets.

The DASH Diet is ranked # 1 overall; it's a balanced diet aimed at preventing and lowering high blood pressure. DASH stands for "Dietary Approaches to Stop Hypertension." By emphasizing fruits, vegetables, whole grains, lean protein, and low-fat dairy it provides potassium, calcium, protein, and fiber, which are needed for fighting high blood pressure. It also stresses cutting back on salt.

Balanced diets are usually best for health and long-term weight control. The DASH Diet is no exception; it also ranked first for healthy eating and diabetes, sixth for heart health, and ninth for short- and long-term weight loss. Importantly, it was also third in the "Easy to Follow" category. U.S. News gave it an overall score of 4.1 out of a possible 5.0. Apparently, no diet is perfect in the eyes of the experts.

In second place, with an overall score of 4.0, was the Therapeutic Lifestyle Change Diet. The TLC Diet plan was created by the National Institutes of Health for the purpose of cutting high cholesterol and promoting cardiovascular health. Interestingly, it was ranked second for heart health, behind the notoriously rigorous Ornish Diet. The TLC Diet is a low-fat version of the DASH Diet. It has no major weaknesses, according to U.S. News. One expert described it as a "very healthful, complete, safe diet."

The Mayo Clinic Diet and the Mediterranean Diet tied for third with combined scores of 3.9. Once again, they resemble the DASH Diet; all three are termed "balanced." Notably, both the Mayo and Med diets strive to make healthy eating a lifelong habit. The Mayo Clinic Diet is aimed at weight loss (where it ranked ninth), with two parts: "Lose it" and "Live it."

What sets the Med Diet apart is that it isn't a *diet* in the usual sense of the word; it's an amalgam of the tastes of people in the countries bordering the Mediterranean Sea. The cultures eating this diet are known for their health and longevity. *U.S. News* lauds the diverse foods and flavors. Fruits, vegetables, whole grains, beans, nuts, legumes, olive oil, and flavorful herbs and spices are all emphasized. Fish is eaten several times a week. Poultry, eggs, cheese, and yogurt are taken in moderation, while sweets and red meat are saved for special occasions. Wine (in moderation) is optional. Physical activity is an important part of the lifestyle.

The aim of the Med Diet, as seen by proponents, is comprehensive in scope. *U.S. News* says it "may include weight loss, heart and brain health, cancer prevention, and diabetes prevention and control." *U.S. News* calls the Med Diet "eminently sensible," adding that the "experts' assessment of it were resoundingly positive, giving this diet an edge over many competitors." (What's not to like?)

Finally, the Weight Watchers Diet is ranked # 5 overall. With the same overall score as the Mayo Clinic and Med diets, it tops the list of the commercial diet plans. Also classified as balanced, *U.S. News* called it "a smart, effective diet." It was the top ranked diet for weight loss.

Regrettably, some high profile diets ended up at the bottom of the list.

The Atkins Diet and the Raw Food Diet tied for 22, with overall scores of 2.3. Ranked 11 among the commercial diet plans, the Atkins Diet didn't stack up with the experts; they agreed that it outperformed most of its competitors for short-term weight loss, but gave it "unfavorable marks" for long-term weight loss, nutrition, safety, and heart health. Readers concurred, with 18,697 saying this diet didn't work for them, compared to 3,699 who said it did. The Raw Food Diet ranked second for both short- and long-term weight loss. The rap against it is that it's "all but impossible" to follow. "Doing it well involves considerable commitment and effort, knowledge, and sacrifice," one expert told *U.S. News*. The Raw Food Diet ranked dead last (# 25) for ease of compliance. Readers voted thumbs down by a 3-to-1 margin.

The Dukan Diet (named for its creator, French physician Pierre Dukan) lined up with the Paleo diet, at the bottom of the rankings, with overall scores of 2.0. The Dukan Diet avows that protein, not calories, is the key to weight loss. You can eat all you want of approved foods—beginning with pure protein—progressing in carefully-defined phases to "Permanent Stabilization." Promising losses of up to 10 pounds in the first week, the

Dukan Diet is loaded down with rules one expert described as "idiotic." (It reminds me of Archie Moore's much ballyhooed pre-fight diet: he chewed meat, extracting the juice, and spit out the rest.) Moreover, "there's no evidence it works," says *U.S. News.* Rated last for heart-health and diabetes, and second only to the Raw Food Diet for ease of compliance, the Dukan Diet, never-theless, garnered 443 favorable votes from readers, compared to only 74 nay sayers.

The Paleo Diet, likewise, occupied the bottom in virtually every category, including weight loss, heart health, diabetes, and nutritional adequacy. The experts were loath to accept that dairy and grains are excluded in the Paleo Diet, saying that puts dieters at risk of missing out on important nutrients. "It's one of the few diets that experts actually considered somewhat unsafe and only somewhat complete nutritionally," U.S. News reported. Readers voted better than 3-to-1 that the diet would not work for them. "A true Paleo Diet might be a great option: very lean, pure meats, lots of wild plants," one expert told *U.S. News.* He quickly added, however, that "duplicating such a regi-men in modern times would be difficult."

Colorado State University Professor (health and exercise sci-ence) Loren Cordain, a leading proponent of the Paleo Diet, was one of several to offer a rebuttal to the negative report from *U.S. News & World Report*: "It is obvious that whoever wrote this piece did not do their homework and has not read the peer reviewed scientific papers which have examined contemporary diets based upon the Paleolithic food groups which shaped the genomes of our ancestors."

U.S. News responded that "the studies were small and short, making strong conclusions difficult."

It's a lot to digest, I know, but well worthwhile. Before you get too far into the decision making process, I want to tell you about some key aspects of the Med Diet.

* * *

As promised, let's talk fish, a mainstay of the Mediterranean Diet—and other benefits of that diet.

A mounting array of evidence shows "that eating more fish is one of the healthiest changes you can make to your diet," *Tufts Health & Nutrition Letter* wrote in a special supplement dated February, 2012.

The 2010 Dietary Guidelines for Americans, I believe for the first time, recognized the health benefits of fish by recommend-ing eating two servings per week, about eight ounces total. Fish deliver lean protein and are good sources of omega-3 fatty acids. This change is especially helpful if fish replace red meat and other foods high in saturated fat. (More about this below) Unfortunately, most Americans eat a minimal amount of fish; and what they do eat is likely to be breaded or deep fried, adding calories and saturated fat.

The best-known connection between fish consumption and health dates from the 1970s, when scientists found a low rate of heart attack in Eskimos eating lots of fish. That led to the realization that omega-3 fatty acids could help protect the heart and arteries. Later research found that omega-3 fats may lower triglycerides, improve blood pressure, prevent blood clots, and reduce heart arrthymia, the leading cause of sudden cardiac death.

Two new studies put participants into groups based on how closely they adhered to an ideal Mediterranean diet. Following up some years later, they calculated the relationship between adherence to the Med Diet and certain disorders, cardiovascular in one study and brain damage in the other.

The first study, published in *The American Journal of Clinical Nutrition* on November 9, 2011, included 2,568 people 69 years of age, give or take 10 years. They found that even modest adherence to the Med Diet may protect against vascular events (stroke, heart attack, and death). Over a follow-up period of nine years, subjects with the highest Med Diet scores had a 33 percent lower risk of vascular death, compared to those with the lowest scores. Moderate alcohol consumption and eating fish containing omega-3 fatty acids and legumes (peas, beans, and lentils), which reduce cholesterol, appeared to have the greatest protective effect against vascular death, according to the study.

"Results support the role of a diet rich in fruit, vegetables, whole grains, fish, and olive oil in the promotion of cardiovascular health," lead author Hannah Gardener and her colleagues concluded.

The second study, published in the February, 2012, *Archives of Neurology*, followed 1,000 people, average age 70. They analyzed the relationship between the Med Diet and damage to small blood vessels in the brain. Using MRI scans, they looked for markers indicating damage to small blood vessels. Such damage can cause small silent strokes with no immediate symptoms, but over time can affect cognitive performance. Hannah Gardener (also the lead researcher in the second study) and her colleagues found that the people with the highest Med Diet scores had the lowest blood vessel damage. Senior researcher Clinton B. Wright, MD, said the study indicates that the Med Diet might be protective of small blood vessels in the brain. More research with more people is needed to be sure, he added.

Another study, described in the *Tufts Letter* special supplement on fish consumption, involved actual brain function. Focusing on only 260 people, average age 70, it was a small study with a big result. About 60% of the participants ate fish at least once a week at the beginning of the study. A repeat survey five years later showed little change in fish consumption. After 10 years, participants underwent an MRI scan to measure their brain volume; five years after that, they had follow-up cognitive testing.

The MRI scans revealed that people eating broiled or baked fish, not fried, on a weekly basis had greater volume in areas of the brain responsible for memory and learning. That was impressive, but the big news was in the cognitive testing. "Only 3.2% of those with the highest fish intake and greatest preservation of gray matter were found to have developed mild cognitive impairment or dementia," the *Tufts Letter* related. "That was in stark contrast to the 30.8% of non-fish eaters who'd suffered cognitive decline." In short, the study suggested that fish consumption reduced the risk of cognitive impairment or dementia by almost 10 times. Now, that is impressive.

While the study had not yet been published in a peer-reviewed journal, lead researcher Cyrus Raji, MD, PhD, of the University of Pittsburg, felt confident enough to conclude: "Consuming baked or broiled fish promotes stronger neurons in the brain's gray matter by making them larger and healthier. This simple lifestyle choice increases the brain's resistance to Alzheimer's disease and lowers risk for the disorder."

* * *

I eat fish four or more times a week and follow a diet much like the Mediterranean Diet. I can tell you first hand that eating that way is filling, satisfying, and easy to follow. *U.S. News* rated the Med Diet # 3 for ease on compliance. The Med-type diet is a delight—and my choice.

Now it's your turn to decide what diet pattern is best for you. Bon Appétit.

* * *

The next section is a logical extension of what we've been talking about. It highlights the need for good fat and how it fits into a healthy eating pattern. An eye-opening discovery has changed the thinking of many on saturated fat, a longtime villain in the eyes of cardiologists and many others. Saturated fat is still considered a problem, but the issue of what to replace it with has come front and center. "Saturated fat is not so bad for you that you can replace it with anything and get benefit," Dr. Dariush Mozaffarian, Brigham and Women's Hospital and Harvard Medical School, told reporters.

"I agree strongly with the notion that rather than focusing on further reductions in saturated fat...we should be thinking much more seriously about finding ways of increasing our intake of polyunsaturated fat," added Dr. Ronald M. Krauss, Children's Hospital Oakland Research Institute, Oakland, California.

Cutting Saturated Fat Alone Not Enough

I have come to appreciate the need for dietary fat more and more over time.

In 1998, my total cholesterol/HDL ratio improved from "very good" to "excellent" after I added a small amount of vegetable oil (olive and then flaxseed) to each of my meals and snacks. My total cholesterol dropped below 200 for the first time in years, perhaps ever. My triglycerides dropped 50 percent, from 153 to 76.

My diet was already low in saturated fat (any kind of fat). I was eating very little processed food. My carbohydrate intake was almost all from whole foods. I thought my diet was just about perfect. But something was missing. That something, it seems, was vegetable oil, which is generally low in saturated fat, and high in mono- and poly-unsaturated fatty acids.

As time went on, I learned about the benefits of omega-3 polyunsaturated fatty acids, found mainly in fatty fish. In 2009, I started taking three fish oil capsules a day, with my main meals. (I was already having salmon several times a week.) My HDL "good" cholesterol skyrocketed to 78. It went from a very good 60 to stunning: 45-70 is the reference range for men.

Slowly but surely, I stopped trying to cut fat, and started striving for an optimum balance of fats. New research suggests that I have been on the right track.

* * *

Two new studies have added more pieces to the good fat-bad fat puzzle. The first one was reported in the *American Journal of Clinical Nutrition* (March 2010). It was a shocker.

Researchers led by Patty W. Siri-Tarino and Ronald M. Krauss analyzed the results of 21 studies involving 347,747 initially healthy participants. During a 5- to 23-year follow-up, 11,006 developed cardiovascular disease. No significant evidence was found that dietary saturated fat is linked to increased risk of heart disease or stroke.

Say what? Saturated fat is okay after all? Think red and processed meat, butter, cheese, ice cream, egg yolk, cookies, and pastries.

Could it be that all of our efforts to cut down on saturated fat were for naught? That would be going too far. Studies have shown that saturated fat can increase LDL "bad" cholesterol, which is a known risk factor for heart disease and stroke. We've been headed in the right direction, but apparently have another lap or two to go.

What we need is more study on what foods should replace saturated fat. The second study explored that issue.

Researchers from Brigham and Women's Hospital and Harvard Medical School (both in Boston) found evidence that replacing saturated fat with polyunsaturated fat does appear to reduce the risk of cardiovascular disease.

That's BIG news! Let's dig into the details and see what we can learn.

The study, led by Dariush Mozaffarian and published March 23, 2010, in the journal *PLoS Medicine*, identified and analyzed the results of eight controlled trials in which 13,614 people replaced dietary saturated fat with polyunsaturated fat for a year or more; mean duration of the studies was 4.25 years. During the course of the trials, participants suffered 1,042 coronary events. Polyunsaturated fat consumption on average accounted for 15 percent of total calories consumed by the intervention participants; among the control groups, polyunsaturated fat accounted for only five percent.

Participants in the intervention groups had a 19% reduced risk of having a coronary event, compared to those in the control groups. Put another way, each 5% increase in the proportion of energy obtained from polyunsaturated fat reduced coronary risk by 10%. Importantly, the researchers also found that the benefits associated with polyunsaturated fat consumption increased in the longer trails; the longer participants stayed on diets high in polyunsaturated fat the more they benefited.

"These findings provide evidence that consuming polyunsaturated fat in place of saturated fat reduces coronary heart disease events," the researchers concluded. "This suggests that rather than trying to lower polyunsaturated fat consumption, a shift toward greater...polyunsaturated fat consumption would significantly reduce rates of coronary heart disease." (Some experts have argued that upping polyunsaturated fat could actually increase heart disease.)

It's important to note that this study did not distinguish between the benefits of *reducing* saturated fat and the benefits of *increasing* polyunsaturated fat. It seems likely that the participants benefited from both dietary changes.

Keep in mind too that polyunsaturated fats come primarily in three forms: nuts, vegetable oils, and fatty fish. Benefits vary and are not fully understood. A mix of all three forms is probably best. (I include all three forms in my diet. My favorite vegetable oil is canola; Carol prefers olive oil.)

Dr. Mozaffarian and Dr. Ronald Krauss (a co-author of the first study) gave us the take-home message.

Krauss concurs that the emphasis should be on replacing saturated fat with polyunsaturated fat. "I agree strongly with the notion that rather than focusing on further reductions in saturated fat...we should be thinking much more seriously about finding ways of increasing our intake of polyunsaturated fat."

"With all the focus on fat and saturated fat and cholesterol, we've put a lot of junk in our diet instead," Dr. Mozaffarian added. "What a person needs to do is to eat the appropriate amount of calories, and eat a healthy, balanced diet."

Dr. Krause elaborated: "An overall eating pattern that emphasizes whole grains rather than refined carbs such as white flour, along with foods high in polyunsaturated fats, such as fish, seeds, nuts, and vegetable oils, is of more value for reducing coronary heart disease risk than simply aiming to further reduce saturated fat."

* * *

With one exception, the diets ranked highest in the *U.S. News* survey were balanced. On the other hand, the diets that didn't fare so well were almost all unbalanced.

Eat a healthy, balanced diet—and exercise. As George Sheehan, a cardiologist and running guru, once wrote, "When you pass on they'll have to beat your heart into submission with a stick."

* * *

Now, let's shift gears and talk about protein. How much do we need to protect and build muscle? Probably less than you've been led to believe; efficient meal planning seems to be the key to insuring that you are getting enough protein.

How Much Protein Can Muscles Use?

How much protein do health-and-fitness minded individuals need? Surprisingly, the answer began taking shape a million or more years ago when we started cooking our food.

Cooking (animal and plant food) made us human, according to *Catching Fire* (Basic Books, 2009), a meticulously researched and persuasive book by Harvard biological anthropologist Richard Wrangham. Now, however, it threatens to wreck our health. Fortunately, there is a simple solution.

Cooking made food softer, easier to digest, taste better, and more energy efficient, allowing us to live on the ground, develop bigger brains, smaller guts, bigger bodies, bonding between males and females, and more. Modern man has taken it another step forward (or backward) with processed food, which makes us fat. Excessive calories from any source, including protein, are in the same category.

Food writer Michael Pollan and others have the right idea, says Professor Wrangham. The answer is to choose *real* food, not *nutrients*. "Real food is natural or only lightly processed, recognizable and familiar," Wrangham explains. "By contrast, nutrients are invisible chemicals, such as essential oils and amino-acids and vitamins, objects of scientific expertise whose significance we must take on faith. The less processed our food, the less intense we can expect the obesity crisis to be," the anthropologist concluded.

That raises the question bodybuilders and others ask over and over. I see it repeatedly in my e-mails. Eddie (not his real name) wrote recently: "I keep carbs low, and fat moderate, [because] I believe that if I don't consume a gram of protein for every pound of bodyweight I will lose muscle mass. I hate to think that drinking protein shakes all day is necessary. That's no way to live!"

Well, Eddie can relax. He doesn't have to live on protein drinks. There is a much more appealing—and healthy—alternative. Ample high-quality dietary protein is required for building and maintaining muscle mass and function, but more is not necessarily better.

A recent study by researchers at the University of Texas Medical Branch at Galveston provides evidence that strongly challenged the idea that high-protein drinks and meat-heavy diets are necessary to preserve and build muscle mass.

The study, led by Douglas Paddon-Jones, PhD, and reported in the September 2009 issue of the *Journal of the American Dietetic Association*, compared muscle synthesis (formation) and anabolic efficiency in response to meals with moderate and high amounts of protein in 17 young (average age 34) and 17 old (average 68 years) volunteers. The subjects were healthy and physically active. Both meals were made up of gently warmed precooked ground beef. One meal contained 30 grams of protein (the rough equivalent of 4 ounces of chicken, fish, dairy, soy, or, in this case, lean beef). The other meal contained three times as much protein, 12 ounces of lean beef and 90 grams of protein.

They had recently demonstrated that a single moderate-size serving of lean beef (4 oz. and 30 grams of protein) increased muscle formation above fasting values by 50% in young and elderly individuals. So that was their baseline measure.

The question they set out to answer was whether more protein would stimulate additional muscle building. "[We] sought to determine whether a three-fold larger protein and energy-rich meal..., representative of the exaggerated portion size available in many restaurants, can be justified by an increased ability to acutely increase muscle protein synthesis in healthy young and elderly individuals."

What they found is instructive. It should put Eddie's mind at rest.

Using blood samples and thigh muscle biopsies, they found no added muscle gain in the subjects eating the larger meal. Young and old volunteers responded the same. "Despite a three-fold increase in protein and energy content, there was no further increase in protein synthesis... in either age group," they reported. "Ingestion of more than 30 g protein in a single meal does not further enhance the stimulation of muscle protein synthesis."

The key finding is that nothing is to be gained by piling on protein in a single meal.

Paddon-Jones and his colleagues suggested that moderate amounts of protein from various sources be consumed over the course of the day. Unfortunately, few Americans follow this advice.

"Usually, we eat very little protein at breakfast, eat a bit more at lunch and then consume a large amount at night," Dr. Paddon-Jones told reporters. "When was the last time you had just 4 ounces of anything during dinner at a restaurant?" he asked. "So we're not taking enough protein on board for efficient muscle-building during the day, and at night we're taking in more than we can use. Most of the excess is oxidized and could end up as glucose or fat."

Paddon-Jones suggested a more efficient and healthy pattern.

"You don't have to eat massive amounts of protein to maximize muscle synthesis, you just have to be a little more clever with how you apportion it," he said. (Are you listening, Eddie?) "For breakfast consider including additional high quality protein. Throw in an egg [see below], a glass of milk, yogurt or add a handful of nuts to get to 30 grams of protein, do something similar to get to 30 for lunch, and then eat a smaller amount of protein for dinner. Do this, and over the course of the day you likely spend much more time synthesizing muscle protein."

* * *

That's great advice. Include some complete protein with each meal and most snacks, and you'll be fine. Forget protein supplements. Stick to whole foods, with all the water and fiber intact. Avoid processed foods, especially those with sugar or fat added. Do this, and you'll get all the protein you can use. What's more, you'll be unlikely to overshoot your calorie needs.

Here's what I'm doing:

Along with mixed whole grains, fruit, and vegetables, my breakfast includes one hard boiled egg—cooking increases the protein value of eggs by about 40 percent—two cups skim milk, and one-fourth cup mixed nuts. I include a like amount of high quality protein in my lunch and evening meal. I also add a little extra protein as soon as possible after workouts.

* * *

We'll end this chapter with two more reasons to consider the Mediterranean-style diet. As you'll recall the Med Diet isn't really a diet; it's a combination of foods favored by populations bordering the Mediterranean Sea. That's an important plus. Foods work together, not in isolation. The new research finds that diet patterns matter, strengthening the case for eating a balanced diet.

Finally, we'll tell you about a recent clinical trial showing why a balanced diet offers the best odds of maintaining weight loss over the long term. Low-fat and low-carbohydrate diets take weight off, but make it difficult to keep it off.

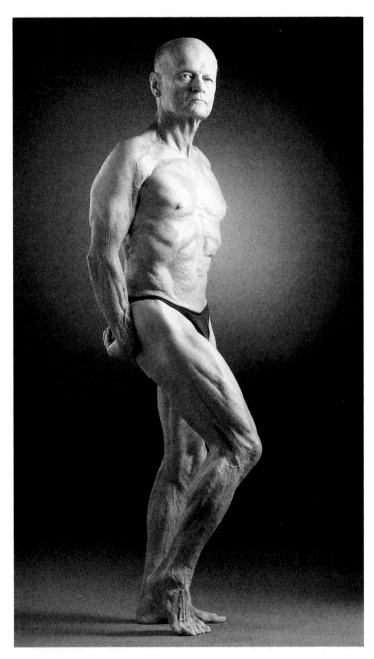

When I was a teenager I consumed so much protein powder that they gave me a discount at the health food store. I got smarter as I grew older. Now I satisfy my protein needs by including some (not a lot) high-quality protein—skim milk, yogurt, egg, fish, and chicken, for example—with most meals or snacks. *Photo by Pat Berrett*

Mediterranean-Style Diet Good for Brain & Heart

Researchers have broadened their investigation beyond individual foods to food patterns. That makes sense; no one eats only one food. We all eat a range of foods which interact. Two new studies compared the effect of two different food combinations—basically a Mediterranean-style diet and a Western-type diet. One study looked at Alzheimer's risk, a limiting factor in brain function. The other looked at heart rate variability, a measure of heart function.

The study on food pattern and Alzheimer's risk was published in the June 2010 issue of *Archives of Neurology*.

Yian Gu, PhD, (Columbia University Medical Center) and colleagues gathered dietary information from 2,148 adults 65 or older living in New York City and followed-up every 18 months for about 4 years.

"We identified a diet pattern strongly associated with lower AD risk," the Gu team explained. "This diet pattern was characterized by higher intakes of salad dressing, nuts, fish, tomatoes, poultry, cruciferous (cabbage family) vegetables, fruits, and dark and green leafy vegetables and a lower intake of high-fat dairy products, red meat, organ meat, and butter."

The low-AD risk pattern strongly resembles a Mediterranean-style diet. The Western-type diet is, of course, often rich in high-fat dairy products, red meat, organ meat, and butter. The report explained several reasons why diet pattern is important, but one cut to the chase: "The effect of a single nutrient or food item may be too small to detect. Indeed, none of the [individual] nutrients was significantly associated with AD risk..."

Although the study wasn't designed to prove cause-and-effect, Gu said, "We controlled for a variety of other lifestyle factors in our analysis, so the relationship between this dietary pattern and Alzheimer's disease could be considered as independent of... smoking, health status, Body Mass Index, etc."

That shows the importance of eating a balanced diet. It also makes it easier to describe and understand the second study, which explains—for the first time—the way in which a Mediterranean-type diet helps reduce the risk of heart disease. The diet pattern included cereal, olive oil, and moderate alcohol consumption; otherwise the Mediterranean-style diet was basically the same as in the first study.

The second study (published online June 15, 2010, in *Circu-*

lation: Cardiovascular Quality and Outcomes) focused on heart rate variability (HRV), an interesting factor you don't hear much about, which makes this study all the more intriguing.

HRV refers to the time interval between heart beats—reduced HRV is a risk factor for coronary artery disease and sudden death. (Less variability is bad; more is good.)

One standard deviation increase in HRV is associated with "24% to 45% lower risk of coronary heart disease death," the researchers explained. In heart attack patients, lower HRV is associated with "at least 2-fold higher risk for all-cause death."

Jun Dai, MD, PhD (assistant professor of nutrition and epidemiology at Indiana University in Bloomington) and her colleagues analyzed the dietary pattern and cardiac data obtained from 276 middle-aged male twins. They scored each participant on how close his food intake correlated with the Mediterranean diet; the higher the score the greater the similarity to a Mediterranean-style diet. A low score indicated a Western-type diet.

To measure HRV, subjects wore an ECG monitor for 24 hours.

The methodology was essentially the same as the Gu study, except using twins allowed the team to gauge the influence of the diet on heart rate variability while controlling for genetic and other familial influences.

"We found that the more an individual's diet conformed to the Mediterranean diet, the greater the heart rate variability, indicating better cardiac autonomic function."

Prior studies had shown an association between individual dietary components and HRV, but this is the first to demonstrate an association between the Mediterranean diet pattern and HRV.

The way (specific physiological effect) the Med-diet reduces the risk of coronary disease has been unknown—until now. (We still don't fully understand the mechanisms linking the Mediterranean diet to HRV.)

The team quantified the change in heart rate variability—and the reduction in risk.

"In our study, the highest quartile of the Mediterranean diet score compared with the lowest quartile was associated with... higher HRV," Dr. Dai and her team reported. "Based on mortality studies, these differences would translate into 9% to 14% reduction in cardiac mortality."

Finally, they capsulized what the study adds that doctors and the rest of us can use: "Whether or not a person has an adverse genetic background or other risk factors for cardiovascular disease, [he or she] would be likely to have better [heart] function if [they follow] a diet similar to the Mediterranean diet."

* * *

A balanced diet such as the Mediterranean diet is also the best way to lose weight and keep it off. New research explains why.

Balanced Diet Keeps Weight Off

Any combination of carbohydrate, protein, and fat that reduces calories below expenditures will take off pounds in the short term. Keeping the pounds off is the problem. A clinical trial published June 27, 2012, in the *Journal of the American Medical Association* concluded that a diet with healthy (whole, unrefined) carbohydrates—rather than low fat or low carbohydrates—does that best.

"Only 1 in 6 overweight and obese adults report ever having maintained weight loss of at least 10% for 1 year," the researchers wrote in introducing the study. "The long term success rates may be even lower," they added. One explanation is loss of motivation. The will to follow a restrictive weight-loss regimen fades over time; people give up and go back to their old eating habits. An alternative explanation, and the one the researchers choose to study, is decline in energy expenditure following weight loss. Our bodies respond to calorie reduction and weight loss by slowing down and making each calorie go farther. Our survival instinct also tells us to eat more.

Led by Cara B. Ebbeling, PhD, and David S. Ludwig, MD, PhD, (associate director and director of the New Balance Foundation Obesity Prevention Center in Boston), the research team measured the drop in energy expenditure that typically follows weight loss and contributes to weight regain. They also monitored changes in specific hormones, fat levels in the blood, and other health markers. Using these determinants, they evaluated the effectiveness of three weight-loss maintenance diets containing equivalent calorie levels.

The first diet—traditionally recommended by the U.S. Government and the American Heart Association—limited fats to 20% of total calories, with 60% carbohydrates, and 20% protein. The second diet, modeled on the Atkins Diet, limited carbohydrate intake to 10% of total calories, with 60% fat and 30% protein. The last diet was low-glycemic, similar to a Mediterranean diet, with 40% carbohydrates, 40% fat, and 20% protein.

The low-glycemic diet is designed to limit blood sugar spikes after eating and, therefore, keep energy and hunger on an even keel. "The low-glycemic index diet aimed to achieve a moderate glycemic load by replacing some grain products and starchy vegetables with sources of healthy fat and low-glycemic vegetables, legumes, and fruits," the researchers wrote. A distinguishing feature of this diet is that refined and easily digested foods are kept to a minimum. (The Atkins-type diet also had a low-glycemic load due to severe restriction of carbohydrates.)

The first step in the study was to put all 21 participants (overweight and obese, age 18 to 40) on a "run-in" diet (45% carbs, 30% fat, and 25% protein) for three months in order to lose 10% to 15% of their bodyweight. The run-in diet was severe, designed to make participants susceptible to gaining the weight back. A month later, the participants began randomly rotating through the three test diets, each for 4 weeks. (All meals were prepared for the participants and intake carefully monitored.)

As you'll see, the final conclusion was a balance of advantages and disadvantages.

The low-fat diet had the biggest (worst) effect on energy expenditure; it also increased triglycerides, a type of fat in the blood, and lowered "good" HDL cholesterol. The low-carb diet, on the other hand, had the least effect on energy expenditures, burning about 300 total calories more per day than those on the low fat diet—only 100 calories fewer than at full weight before the loss. Unfortunately, the positive results came at a cost—increases in cortisol, a hormonal measure of stress, and C-reactive protein (CRP), a measure of inflammation. "Higher cortisol levels may promote adiposity, insulin resistance, and cardiovascular disease," Ebbeling et al explained. CRP is an independent risk factor for developing heart disease.

Those on the low-glycemic diet were in the middle, with energy burn about 150 calories a day more than those on the low-fat diet. Importantly, the good news on energy expenditure (compare to the low-fat dieters) came without any negative impact on blood fats, stress, or inflammation. On balance, that made it the best of the three diets for losing weight and keeping it off.

The researchers summarized their findings: "The very low-carbohydrate diet had the most beneficial effect on energy expenditure..., but this restrictive regimen may increase cortisol excretion and CRP. The low-glycemic index diet appears to have qualitatively similar, although smaller, metabolic benefits to the very low-carbohydrate diet, possibly without the deleterious effects of physiological stress and chronic inflammation. These findings suggest that a strategy to reduce glycemic load rather than dietary fat may be advantageous for weight-loss maintenance and cardiovascular disease prevention."

The low-glycemic diet also had the advantage of being more user-friendly.

"In addition to the benefits noted in the study, we believe that low-glycemic-index diets are easier to stick to on a day-to-day basis, compared to low-carb and low-fat diets, which many people find limiting," Dr. Ebbeling told e Science News. "Unlike low-fat and very-low-carbohydrate diets, the low-glycemic-index diet doesn't eliminate entire classes of food, likely making it easier to follow and more sustainable."

Put another way, a balanced diet is more satisfying and easier to follow over the long term. That makes it much easier to keep weight off.

* * *

According to the Ebbeling-Ludwig study, continuation of the low-fat diet (high in carbohydrates) would require about an hour of additional moderate-intensity exercise each day in order to keep the weight off. That and loss of the satiety value of fatty food (fish, vegetable oil, nuts, and an occasional dessert) would likely lead to regain. On the other hand, sticking with the low-carb diet would likely produce a practically irresistible craving for carbohydrates, along with an increased risk of developing heart disease and diabetes.

That leaves the more satisfying—and healthy—low-glycemic diet that might require a little more physical activity. Most people can benefit from a little more exercise anyway. Sounds like a win-win to me.

* * *

The Ebbeling-Ludwig study is a perfect lead-in to the next chapter, on new discoveries in dieting and weight loss. It's a topic that has puzzled and frustrated nearly everyone at one time or another. The new findings take many of the mysteries out of weight control. If you know what to expect, good and not so good, your odds of reaching your ideal weight—and staying there—will be far greater.

Chapter Ten

Dieting Dynamics

Weight Loss Is a Dynamic Process— Not a Straight Line

"This research helps us understand why one person may lose weight faster or slower than another, even when they eat the same diet and do the same exercise," said Kevin D. Hall, PhD, referring to a study reported in an issue of *Lancet* devoted to obesity (August 27, 2011).

Government budget projections are notoriously inaccurate because they use static analysis. For example, they assume that a 10 percent tax increase will produce 10 percent more revenue. It almost never works out that way. People adapt, they are dynamic; they change their behavior when taxes go up. Tax something and you almost always get less of it. Diets are the same. They almost never work out as planned. Our bodies adjust to energy deficits created by dieting or exercise in different ways.

Researchers at the National Institutes of Health have created a mathematical model of what happens when people of varying weights, diets, and exercise habits try to change their weight. The results have the potential to change our perspective on weight control. The more we understand about the process, the more realistic we are, the happier we're likely to be with our results. Aligning expectations and reality can make us better stewards of our bodies.

To test and fine tune the model, Kevin D. Hall and colleagues compared projected weight changes to actual changes in real people. Several important insights emerged: 1) Steady weight loss is a myth, 2) Heavier people respond faster to diet change than people with less initial body fat, and 3) We can predict the long-term effect of a single permanent change in diet or exercise for the average overweight person.

The basic principle of bodyweight change is that you must tip the balance between energy intake and expenditure. Tip it one way and you gain weight and tip it the other way and you lose weight. What could be simpler than that? Sounds straightforward; unfortunately, it's not.

The widely quoted *3500 calories per pound rule* is a well-meaning myth. "This ubiquitous weight loss rule was derived by estimation of the energy content of weight loss [3500 calories in a pound of fat]," Hall et al wrote, "but it ignores dynamic physiological adaptations to altered body weight that lead to changes of both resting metabolic rate as well as the energy cost of physical activity." Put another way, negative calorie imbalance—through diet or exercise—causes the body to slow down and operate more frugally and efficiently over time.

While it is generally recognized that the static weight loss rule is simplistic, little has been done to measure how diet and exercise translate into weight loss over time. Hall and his team addressed this issue by using a mathematical model that incorporates our knowledge of how the human body responds to changes in diet and physical activity.

Let's examine the key variables.

Body fat contains about five times more energy (calories) than lean tissue. That's bound to affect weight loss, but how? People with a higher proportion of body fat lose body weight at a different rate than those with a lower percentage of fat. "People with a higher initial adiposity partition a greater proportion of a net energy imbalance towards gain or loss of body fat versus lean tissue than do people with low initial adiposity," the Hall team wrote. Simply put, a greater proportion of weight loss is fat for people who start out with more fat. As you become leaner, however, the rate of fat loss slows down. Frustrating as that may seem, it makes sense; there's a good reason for the shift.

While the underlying mechanism is complex and not fully understood, we've known the outcome for many years. "The net result can be described by a simple equation first presented more than 30 years ago and subsequently updated and validated," the researchers wrote.

We know that the relative value of lean and fat tissues is dynamic; it changes as weight loss progresses. As the body becomes leaner, fat becomes more important for survival and thus more valuable, while the value of lean tissue declines.

These factors have been incorporated in a mathematical model. Actual weight loss studies provide validation of the model. Notably, the data from the studies was not available when the model was being developed. So the model has stood the test of time.

Let's see how it would work in hypothetical cases.

The Hall report predicted the results of putting a 220-pound sedentary man on a diet that cut calories by a steady 480 per day and gave him 10 years to lose weight. What would happen? They predicted that his bodyweight would plateau at about 165 pounds, with roughly half of the weight loss in the first year, and 95% of the loss in three years. The last 5% was predicted to come off over that last seven years!

Even well-read dieters are likely to be surprised by that prediction. The popular diet rule (3500 calories per pound) would predict that a steady daily 480-calorie reduction would result in a loss of 48.5 pounds in the first year, which is almost 100% greater than the model would predict; the model predicted about 27.5 pound in the first year.

After the first year, the model predicts that the rate of loss would slow by half over the next two years, that is, the loss would be another 27.5 pounds over those years. As indicated above, at the three year mark calorie intake and expenditure would come into virtual balance over the final seven years, dropping only a few more pounds.

Keep in mind that the model reflects only one permanent change in diet: a steady daily calorie reduction of 480; everything else was unchanged. There is no change in energy expenditure, no added exercise.

It's probably wouldn't happen that way in real life, but the general course should be roughly the same. For one thing, perfect adherence is rare—how many people would cut calories by 480 every day for three years, much less 10 years?

As noted earlier, body composition would also make a difference. Adults with a higher—or lower—percentage of body fat would be expected to lose more—or less—weight for the same reduction in energy intake.

A fatter man might go down to 155 pounds, but most of the loss would probably still be in the first three years. A leaner man might plateau at 175 pounds, because the lean tissue mass is preserved.

Keep in mind, too, that the bodyweight time course is dynamic; it changes as the fat-to-lean ratio changes. As the body becomes leaner, fat becomes more important for survival and the value of lean tissue declines. The leaner you become, the more difficult it becomes to lose fat.

What about physical activity? What if our reference man only increased physical activity by 480 calories every day? Does an increase in physical activity necessarily lead to the same weight loss as an energy-equivalent decrease in food intake? Not necessarily, according to the researchers. Again using a 220-pound sedentary overweight man, the Hall team compares cutting calories by 480 per day (the first model) with increasing activity by a like amount (the second model).

"Such a relatively modest increase of physical activity results in slightly more rapid and greater predicted weight loss...," Hall et al wrote. "However, as the magnitude of each intervention

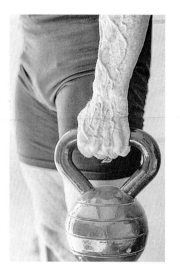

Becoming lean and muscular takes patience and persistence. You must lose weight very slowly to avoid setting off survival mechanisms that slow fat loss and cannibalize muscle.
Photo by Laszlo Bencze

increases, there is a point when diet leads to greater weight loss than does physical activity." That's because the energy expenditure of added physical activity is proportional to bodyweight itself, the researchers explained. As bodyweight goes down a fixed amount of exercise burns fewer calories.

That makes sense, doesn't it?

* * *

The take away message from these studies should be a positive one. When you decide to lose weight, remember that the process is not a straight line—give yourself some time, and be kind to yourself as the process unfolds. Amass more self-knowledge. Be smart with your efforts. If the model shows what happens with only one change (calories), the results with two variables (calories and exercise) are almost sure to produce better results.

I believe that a *slight* decrease in calories combined with a *slight* increase in physical activity is the best plan. It's easier on you and doesn't set off metabolic alarm bells in your body. As I wrote in *Ripped 3*, bigger changes in calories or activity "defeat your purpose in three ways: 1) your metabolism slows down to save energy; 2) you lose muscle tissue; and 3) you get hungry and binge."

Creating an eating and exercise plan that you can live with comfortably on a daily, monthly, and yearly basis is the smart way to achieve your goal of having a lean and fit body.

* * *

Scientists have a single rule of thumb for weight loss. Here's what they say:

"Every permanent change in energy intake of 10 calories per day will lead to an eventual weight change of about one pound, and it will take about one year to achieve half of the total weight change and 95% of the total weight change will result in about 3 years."

So a permanent reduction of 10 calories will lead to a loss of one pound in three years—and 200 calories would take off 20 pounds. That doesn't sound like much, I know, but taking 20 pounds off and keeping it off can be a life-changing achievement.

Here's how I suggest putting the rule-of-thumb into action.

* * *

If your goal is to lose 50 pounds, the formula says you will need to create a steady daily energy deficit of 500 calories (10 x 50). The best way to do that is to reduce calorie intake by 250 and increase physical activity by a like amount. That way your fat cells will notice the difference, but you probably won't. (Avoid the temptation to cut more severely.)

Do that consistently and you'll lose about 25 pounds the first year and the second 25 pounds over the next two years. You'll lose the full 50 pounds in about 3 years. (It took you longer than that to put the weight on, and you should expect to take a while losing it.) That would be a terrific result, accomplished with little, if any, discomfort. What's more, you won't be tempted to regain the weight. Continue eating sensibly and exercising regularly and you'll be lean for life.

Some people will lose faster and others slower, but almost everyone should be successful on this plan. If you're eating the typical American diet of mostly processed foods with lots of sugar and salt added, a switch to a balanced diet of whole or minimally processed foods will put you on track to meet your goal without suffering. You won't even have to count calories. (I never do.) Add two days a week of aerobic exercise and two days of resistance training, and stay active in between workouts and you'll be amazed at how much better you'll look and feel.

Be smart. Be patient. Be successful!

* * *

Now, let's take a look at food instincts that—like the survival system embedded in the weight loss model—kept us alive in prehistoric times. Fortunately, these instincts can be made to work for us today. You'll be surprised how easy it is when you understand how to work with—rather than against—your food instincts.

Managing Food Instincts

"Spiders spin webs because they are spiders, and we humans eat the way we do and like the foods we do because we're humans," Susan B. Roberts, PhD, wrote in *The Instinct Diet* (Workman, 2008). That's our survival instincts at work.

Weight loss from diets—all kinds—often stop after six months. At two years the dieters in a recent study (February 26, 2009, *New England Journal of Medicine*) had regained half the loss and were on the way to regaining the entire loss. (Keep in mind that the weight loss model discussed above assumes perfect compliance.)

"The effect of any particular diet....was minuscule, but the effect of individual behavior is humongous," said Frank M. Sacks, MD, lead author of the study and a professor at the Harvard School of Public Health.

Dr. Susan Roberts, professor of nutrition and psychiatry at Tufts University, has studied basic food instincts—running a research laboratory for 17 years—which control how we eat. She has found "striking agreement" that five things affect our eating behavior: hunger, availability, variety, familiarity, and how rich or calorie-dense the food is.

We cannot override these instincts. But once we understand the signals that trigger them, we can make our instincts work for us, not against us.

Let's look at how they work one by one—and how we can work with them.

HUNGER: The solution is to acknowledge—and accept—that we need to satisfy our hunger. Stop fighting it. We like feeling full.

Roberts says there are four effective ways to control our need to feel full: high-fiber, high-protein, low-Glycemic Index, and volume. She recommends using them all; that's important, you'll need all four methods to stay satisfied.

It's well-known that fiber in the diet makes you feel full. Roberts recommends including high fiber foods (grains, cereal, beans, vegetables, fruits) in most meals. "Do be sure to drink six to eight glasses of water daily when you eat more fiber," she counsels, "to get the full benefits and prevent constipation." It's the water-holding property that makes fiber so filling. (Water, of course, takes up space but contains no calories.)

Foods high in protein, such as fish or chicken, are also very satisfying, and slow the return of hunger. They are digested

165

slowly and don't cause large fluctuations in blood sugar. Unlike many carbohydrate sources, protein foods are digested over hours rather than minutes. Roberts suggests combining fish or chicken with green vegetables or salad. "The trouble with high-protein diets," she warns, "is that they can get really boring... The temptation to cheat may get stronger and stronger."

That's why she suggests making high-protein one of many options. "You can go to a restaurant and have half a lean entrée with a side salad and a glass of mineral water and keep your diet without making a public fuss about it." (Carol and I frequently split an entrée when eating out; we almost always go away feeling full and satisfied.)

Low-glycemic foods, which cause only a small rise in blood sugar, are another good option for controlling how much we eat. "Low-GI foods have been shown to suppress hunger extremely well," Roberts explained, "because the more stable blood glucose produced by these foods tells our food brain that all is well and we don't need to eat again yet."

Confused about what foods are low-glycemic? Roberts has the answer: "Here's how to think about it: Unrefined, whole, chunky, lightly cooked and sour foods almost always have the low GIs."

Another alternative is combining low-GI foods with high-GI foods for taste. Roberts wrote, "Low-GI foods, when eaten alone, may not taste as good as foods with higher GI values. They're digested more slowly, so our brain learns to like them but not love them, probably because they don't release as many of the feel-good taste and reward chemicals."

A steady diet of low-GI foods will tempt you to cheat, Roberts warned. "We...seem to instinctively crave carbohydrates, and any plan that doesn't have a way to give you some carbs in a healthy form will be fundamentally unsatisfying after a while." (The brain's primary fuel is glucose (blood sugar), which is supplied mainly by carbohydrates in the diet.)

The fourth and last way to deal with hunger is volume. Pioneered by *Volumetrics* author Barbara Rolls, this method of controlling hunger relies on the fact that volume trumps calories in making us feel full. "The mechanism isn't known for sure," Roberts explained, "but is probably related to the activation of stretch receptors in the stomach or simply our perception of the *right* amount of food. As long as food is bulky, it doesn't matter as much where the majority of calories come from."

Good high-volume options are high-fiber cereal with low-fat

milk, soup with dense particles to slow down digestion, and large dinner-size salads with something substantial on top, such as grilled chicken breast, seeds, or nuts. Something chewy is good, because chewing helps to make you feel full and satisfied.

Remember, don't pick one or two ways to cope with the hunger instinct, use all four (fiber, protein, low-GI, and volume) to make sure every meal or snack makes you feel full and satisfied—without overloading you with calories.

We've given lots of details on managing the hunger instinct, because hunger can't be ignored; satisfaction is the only way to overcome it. Hunger is clearly *the* basic food instinct. Dealing with it puts us well on the way to controlling the other four instincts, which we'll cover briefly.

AVAILABILITY: This one is pretty straightforward. If food is there, we're programmed to eat it. It's the basis for my practice of putting on the table only the food I plan to eat. If I want more, I get up and get it—but I stop and think about it first. I almost always decide I've had all I *really* want. That simple rule has saved me from eating many thousands of excess calories.

Dr. Roberts tells us that this instinct came into being eons ago. "This was essential for survival, and the most successful survivors were those who ate whenever food was available."

"So it's up to you to avoid temptation by getting rid of what tempts you," Roberts wrote. It's as simple as that. Get the bad stuff out of your home—and don't buy more. If you really crave an ice cream sundae or a deep dish pizza, go out and have it. Just don't bring it home, and don't make a habit of it.

CALORIE DENSITY: Those who have read my first book, *Ripped*, will remember my cardinal rule: "Avoid concentrated calories." I discovered that by eating only whole, unprocessed foods, you avoid almost all concentrated calorie foods, and you won't overeat.

That's still my rule.

"Almost everybody loves high-calorie foods, but does this mean we're *instinctively* attracted to foods that are jam-packed with calories?" Roberts asked rhetorically. "You bet it does," she answered.

Again, it goes back to ancient times. "An affinity for foods loaded with calories was an asset during early human development, when the next meal was an unpredictable event," Roberts explained. "The more calories per ounce a food has, the more we prefer it."

Macronutrients don't seem to matter, says Roberts. "In fact, the most popular foods are actually a mixture of [carbs, fat and protein]...Our strongest preferences are for foods containing some of those rapidly digested white carbs, with a little fat and protein thrown in for good measure."

Attempting to avoid calorie dense food altogether is not a good idea, however. It won't work. The key is to recognize the danger and be careful not to overdo.

An occasional splurge can actually be beneficial, because it gets the craving out of your system, allowing you to happily go back to healthy eating most of the time. The second part, what you eat most of the time is, of course, the key.

FAMILIARITY: My practice of eating frequent meals and snacks to stay ahead of the hunger curve—and in control— dovetails with this instinct. I could just as easily make a habit of skipping breakfast, snacking haphazardly during the day, and stuffing myself in the evening—but it wouldn't help me control how much I eat.

The same is true of the kind of food we usually eat. You can make a habit of eating healthy meals, or Coke, burgers and fries.

"Instinctively, we're drawn to what we know," Roberts explained. "Historically, this instinct kept us safe. For our Paleolithic ancestors, being cautious about trying new foods was all that stood between a good dinner and death by poison."

You can change, however. Start eating healthy, regular meals and pretty soon you'll get used to it—and actually prefer eating that way.

"Learn to love what's good for you," Roberts suggested. "Repetition is all it takes." Try it. You'll like it.

VARIETY: We are programmed to eat widely. Again, it was a matter of survival. "Because no single food has all the nutrients that humans need, it was essential for them to eat a wide variety of foods in order to get the healthy nutrition that would keep them alive," Roberts related. "Variety *instinctively* felt right."

Like the other food instincts, this one can work for or against us.

Too much variety leads to overeating. "Even fish and other wild creatures eat more food when they're presented with more variety," Roberts wrote. "In study after study, variety has been shown to have a huge effect on the amount of food we eat."

This instinct is closely related to the availability instinct. The difference is that availability relates to amount, and variety relates to, well, variety. The key is to understand that both instincts are in play.

168

Not surprisingly, the fixes are much the same. Variety can be good if it's the right kind. Roberts and her colleagues at the Tufts lab discovered that eating a wide variety of high calorie foods leads to weight gain. Conversely, eating a wide variety of vegetables can double or triple total vegetable consumption, which reduces overall calorie intake.

So the answer to both instincts is to replace the bad stuff with the good stuff. A wide variety of junk food is likely to make you fat, but a house with lots of fruits, vegetables, whole grains, beans, fish, seeds, and nuts will help you become and stay lean.

* * *

Let's turn to some little understood concepts that can make a big difference in how well we manage our weight. We'll start with the effect of exercise on appetite and how our gut says *I'm full*.

Exercise Curbs Appetite— Our Gut Brain Does the Same

Exercise makes our appetite control mechanism work better. People who don't exercise are more likely to fall victim to creeping obesity; they eat a little more than they need, and the fat slowly piles up on their body.

We've long known that exercise helps control eating and fat gain, but we are only now beginning to learn the details of how it works. Brazilian researchers at the University of Campinas in Sao Paulo are helping us understand the underlying mechanism.

Their study, reported in the August, 2010, *PLoS Biology*, is long and complicated, with an amazing number of charts and graphs, but the bottom line is straightforward: Exercise makes the brain more sensitive to key chemicals that signal when we've had enough to eat. (The study involved rodents. That's where the learning usually begins; we can't dissect the brains of humans.)

Simply put, exercise made the rodent's hypothalamus better able to interpret hormonal signals of fullness.

This next part is important to a full understanding of how exercise affects appetite.

"Our study shows that acute exercise per se did *not* evoke any meaningful effect, in terms of food intake in lean animals," the researchers reported, "but interestingly, it was crucial for suppressing hyperphagia [overeating]" in obese animals with impaired hypothalamic insulin and leptin signaling.

In short, *if it ain't broke exercise won't fix it.* For fat animals—and perhaps humans—who need it, however, exercise can be a Godsend.

Exercise has long been considered a mainstay of weight control, but only now are studies such as this uncovering the full benefits. Exercise not only increases calorie burn, it also regulates and, if necessary, improves communications between the gut and the brain.

That brings us to the appetite control cops in our digestive system.

"Your Stomach Really Does Have a Mind of Its Own," *The Wall Street Journal* headlined a "Personal Journal" feature by Gautam Naik (January 25, 2011).

Millions of nerve cells in our esophagus, stomach, small intestine, and colon operate as an appetite-control second brain. These digestive track neurons talk together and with brain cells in the cranium—about fullness. "This gut brain helps to control muscular contractions and gut secretions," Naik reported. "It also balances the body's hunger and satiety, or feelings of fullness, and communicates those states to the big brain."

"The body is in a state of continual hunger—its default position," Naik continues. "But several factors work to curtail the hunger instinct, such as the presence of food in the digestive track, or the flow of nutrients in the blood. When these satiety factors dissipate, the body again demands food."

Naik describes three key systems in our gut brain that tell our big brain when it's time to stop eating. Understanding how they work allows us to help them do their job more effectively.

Stomach Stretching: As food fills the stomach, it stretches, and the gut brain sends a neural message to the big brain: *Getting crowded down here—stop eating.* That's why it's important to avoid refined and sugary foods, which are dense with calories and don't take up much room. Whole foods—especially fruits, vegetables and whole grains—fill the stomach without overshooting calorie needs.

Peptide Release: The gut brain also senses when there are nutrients in the gastrointestinal tract and releases peptides into the blood, sending another fullness signal to the big brain. Peptides are usually formed when proteins are digested in the gut. This presents another opportunity to make the system work in our favor. Including high quality protein in meals (eggs, fish and chicken are good examples) helps us feel full with fewer calories.

Ileal Brake: This mechanism also involves peptide release.

The ileum is the lower part of the small intestine. The ileal brake sends an *I'm full* message to the big brain when fat reaches the ileum. That's why it's a good idea to include some healthy fat in each meal; olive oil, nuts, and fish are good sources. Fat slows digestion and puts the brake on appetite.

In short, whole foods, quality protein, and healthy fat in meals help your gut do a better job telling you when it's time to stop eating.

* * *

We are born to be active—and lean. Our gut brain reflects millions of years of evolution. Obesity had no place in a world where we had to chase down our dinner and move with the seasons to survive. Exercising and eating wisely maximize our chances of realizing our birthright. Help your body and it will help you.

* * *

The next section makes a point that every dieter needs to know.

It's the Body Fat that Matters

When you step on the bathroom scale, the weight you see isn't the whole story. What's missing is how much is fat and how much is muscle, your body composition. That's old news to most fitness-minded people, but it's something that everyone needs to know. It's a key point in an important study about diet and weight control. When it comes to fat gain, the new study says, it's how much you eat, not what you eat, that counts. You might never know it, however, if you go by weight gain alone.

Excess calories are what matters when it comes to fat gain. If you eat too much—carbohydrate, fat, or protein—you will gain fat. The new finding is that a deficiency in protein makes matters worse. Short-change protein, eating the same number of calories, and you will not gain as much weight. But you will gain just as much fat as you would have if you had eaten adequate protein.

The study is the latest in a long line challenging the concept that manipulating macronutrients (carbohydrate, fat, and protein) is the secret to weight control.

Some researchers maintain that diets low or high in protein are less metabolically efficient and, therefore, produce less weight gain. In other words, low or high protein diets are said to make the body work harder, which means there won't be as many excess calories. So you won't gain as much weight.

Dr. George A. Bray and his colleagues designed a study to test this assertion under tightly controlled and randomized conditions. Based on earlier findings, they anticipated that a diet high in protein would lead to less weight gain. (They were in for a surprise.)

They fed 25 young men and woman 1,000 excess calories daily for eight weeks, varying the proportion of protein and fat. Participants were randomly divided to diets containing low (5%), normal (15%), and high (25%) protein. All meals were taken in strictly controlled conditions; participants lived in the metabolic ward of an inpatient research center. Carbohydrates were held steady at 41% to 42% of calories, while fat intake varied with protein content. Participants were monitored to make sure they ate all the food they were given.

The basic menu was the same for all participants. Protein sources included turkey, chicken, tuna, and pork chops. Tuna salad provides an example of how protein intake was controlled. The low protein group received more mayonnaise and less tuna, while the high protein group got more tuna and less mayonnaise; the normal protein group split the difference.

The surprising results:

The low-protein diet group gained significantly less weight: 7 pounds compared to 13 pounds for the normal protein group, and 14 pounds for the high-protein group. Importantly, body fat increased practically the same in all three groups: 8.07 lbs, 7.62 lbs, and 7.59 lbs, respectively. Change in lean body mass, however, differed significantly; it went *down* 1.54 lbs in the low-protein group, and *up* 6.33 lbs and 7.02 lbs, in the normal and high protein groups, respectively.

"In summary, weight gain when eating a low protein diet (5% of energy from protein) was blunted compared with weight gain when eating a normal protein diet (15% of energy from protein) with the same number of extra calories," the researchers concluded. "*Calories alone, however, contributed to the increase in body fat.* In contrast, protein contributed to the change in energy expenditure and lean body mass, *but not to the increase in body fat.*" (Emphasis mine)

"The body was confronted with excess calories, but it didn't care where they came from," Dr. Bray, a researcher at Pennington Biomedical Researcher in Baton Rouge, Louisiana, said. "The only thing it can do is put them into fat."

It's calories that build fat. That's important to know; excess weight and obesity are growing problems all over the world. It makes no difference whether you eat carbs, fat, or protein; if you eat too much, you're going to get fat. That's the first lesson.

Another important message is that protein content does matter. Those eating 15% or 25% protein gained lean muscle mass along with the fat. That's a good thing, because more muscle means faster metabolism. The problem is that the diet low in protein caused a decrease in lean body mass.

"There is no health-related benefit to a reduction in lean body mass," Dr. Bray observed. That's a bit of an understatement because, by slowing metabolism, lower lean body mass encourages further weight gain. An editorial that accompanied the report of the study in the January 4, 2012, *Journal of the American Medical Association* focused on the negative effect of overeating beyond weight gain.

The editorial by Zhaoping Li, MD, PhD, and David Heber, MD, PhD, Center for Human Nutrition at the David Geffen School of Medicine at UCLA, emphasized that body weight gain may underestimate the hazards of the Western diet, which tends to be high in fat and carbohydrates and low in protein. As shown in the Bray study, that diet (low protein) causes fat gain that doesn't show up on your bathroom scale. "Accumulation of excess fat is associated with obesity related conditions, whereas increased muscle mass is beneficial because of its positive effect on metabolism," Li and Heber explained. "Humans are better adapted to starvation with subsequent maintenance of lean body mass than they are to overfeeding, which results in body fat accumulation," they added.

Gaining fat and losing lean body mass—which the typical American does as he or she grows older—is a prescription for disaster. On the bright side, "it is possible for patients who exercise and eat adequate protein to build lean body mass," Li and Heber counseled. "Because muscle weighs more than fat per unit of volume, it is possible for patients to gain weight with muscle mass while reducing waist circumference and intra-abdominal fat."

You can gain muscle and lose fat at the same time, a change that shows up in the mirror and how your clothes fit—but not on the scale. That's a message doctors should be giving their patients.

At minimum, doctors (and everyone else) should look beyond body weight. "The goals for obesity treatment should involve fat reduction rather than simple weight loss, along with a better understanding of nutritional science," Li and Heber concluded.

Specifically, doctors should warn their patients about the hazards of eating a diet high in calories and low in protein.

* * *

All of this comes down to three simple *Don'ts*: 1) Don't neglect protein intake (don't overdo it either), 2) Don't be taken in by complicated and onerous macronutrient formulas, and 3) Don't overeat.

* * *

The next section is about a practice that has worked for me over decades. I believe in making small reductions in calorie intake so that your fat cells notice, but you don't. That makes it easier to stick to your eating plan. It's no-suffering dieting at its best.

Small Calorie Reduction, Large Weight Change

A new study from the Division of Nutritional Sciences at Cornell University in Ithaca, NY, shows that small calorie reductions leading to weight loss go unnoticed.

The mechanism illustrated may be the most powerful tool in the weight-control tool box. It's a little appreciated—and very important—key to losing weight and keeping it off.

Seventeen volunteers ate all meals and snacks from food provided by the researchers from Monday through Friday for five consecutive weeks. For the first week, all participants selected food from a buffet where each food was weighed before and after eating. Participants were allowed to eat whatever they wanted. This allowed the researchers to measure the total—and unrestricted—amount consumed each day.

For the next two weeks, half of the group selected their lunch from one of six commercially available portion-controlled meals; each lunch contained the same number of calories. They were allowed to eat as much as they wanted at other meals or snacks. For the last two weeks (four and five), the other half choose from the potion-controlled lunches. Food intake was closely monitored throughout the study. Bodyweight was also carefully monitored.

Consuming the portion-controlled lunches reduced consumption by 250 calories per day.

"More importantly," the two researchers wrote, "no sign of calorie compensation was evident across the 10 days of testing, an observation substantiated by a significant loss of body weight." Participants were free to eat more after eating the calorie-reduced lunches, but they didn't.

In confirmation, participants lost, on average, 1.1 pounds during the two weeks of calorie-reduced lunches. The correlation between energy intake and weight loss was "highly significant," the researchers reported.

Interestingly, measures of hunger taken before consumption of the smaller lunch did not change over the 10 testing sessions despite an increasing cumulative energy deficit. There was also no change in hunger prior to dinner following the smaller lunch.

What's more, the weight loss suggests that the participants didn't overeat on weekends. There was no significant weight change from Friday to Monday. Moreover, there was no change in hunger ratings from Friday to Monday.

"The results suggest that the mere substitution of one smaller meal each day is sufficient to cause reduction in daily energy intake and a significant amount of weight," the co-authors concluded.

Over a year, a loss of 1.1 pound every two weeks would total over 25 pounds—without feeling the need to compensate by eating more to make up the lunchtime calorie reduction. (As we saw earlier in this chapter, the body adapts to calorie reduction, so the rate of reduction may decline over time.)

What's the explanation?

"It seems that the reduction in *total daily energy* occurs because humans fail to accurately compensate for the reduced energy of the meal replacements by increasing intake at succeeding meals, at least over a period of 10 successive days of measurement," the authors wrote. Apparently, humans do not regulate energy intake with any precision. We don't miss small daily calorie reductions.

* * *

This approach works for me. It will work for you as well. Remember, small calorie reductions, consistently, over time, produce large weight reductions. I know, it sounds too simple, too easy, too painless, but it does work.

(The study was published in the October, 2011, issue of the journal *Appetite*. Doctoral student Carly Pacanowski co-authored the study with Cornell professor David A. Levitsky.)

* * *

You've probably heard it said that breakfast is the most important meal of the day. Well, it's true for many reasons, but especially so for those trying to manage their calorie intake.

Hearty Breakfast More Important than Calories

Researchers from Israel found that eating a high-carbohy-drate, high-protein breakfast overcomes the hunger and craving that lead to long-term weight gain. Dieters who ate a hearty breakfast lost several times as much weight as dieters who ate the same number of calories, but skimped on breakfast.

The details—and the explanation—are eye-opening.

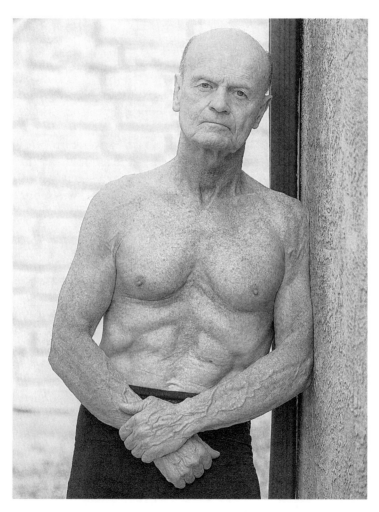

I eat a balanced diet of whole or minimally processed foods—and cut back slightly before photos or other special occasions. It works for me and it will work for you. *Photo by Laszlo Bencze*

One hundred and ninety-three obese men and women were randomly assigned to one of two diet groups with identical calorie intake; the men ate 1600 calories a day and the women 1400. The difference was that one group ate a low carbohydrate breakfast containing 300 calories and the other group ate a 600 calorie breakfast high in carbohydrate and protein. The 600 calorie breakfast included a sweet snack; participants were allowed to select chocolate, cookies, cake, etc. (The sweet snacks were overkill to make an important point; see below.)

In addition to weight loss and maintenance, the researchers compared the effect of the two breakfasts on appetite, craving, and ghrelin levels. (Ghrelin is a hormone that increases hunger.)

Halfway into the 32 week study, both groups had lost about the same amount of weight: 33 pounds in the skimpy breakfast group and 30 pounds in the hearty breakfast group. Again, both groups consumed the same number of calories. What happened next is startling.

During the second 16 weeks, the men and women given the low-carbohydrate, low-calorie breakfast regained an average of 22 pounds per person, while the high-carb, high-protein breakfast group lost another 15 pounds. At the end of the study, those consuming the 600 calorie breakfast lost an average of 34 pounds more than those who were limited to 300 calories at breakfast, 45 pounds compared to a net loss of only 11 pounds.

Importantly, ghrelin, the hunger hormone, rose before every meal, but was reduced 45.2% after the high-carb, high-protein breakfast, compared to only 29.5% after the low-carb, low-calorie breakfast. "Satiety was significantly improved and hunger and craving scores significantly reduced" in the group that ate the 600 calorie breakfast, the researchers reported.

Though they consumed the same daily calories, "the participants in the low carbohydrate diet group had less satisfaction, and felt that they were not full," lead researcher Professor Daniela Jakubowicz explained, noting that their cravings for sugar and carbohydrate were more intense and eventually caused them to cheat on the diet plan. "But the group that consumed a bigger breakfast, including dessert, experienced few if any cravings for those foods later in the day."

"To achieve long term weight loss, the diet meal timing and macronutrient composition has to counteract mechanisms that encourage regain after weight loss," the researchers from Tel Aviv University and Hebrew University in Jerusalem wrote in summary.

"Enriched breakfast may be a strategy to maintain weight loss and prevent regain over time," they added. Satisfying cravings is a better strategy for weight loss success than deprivation.

The full study was reported in the journal *Steroids* on March 10, 2012. (The study was also reported in *Science Daily*.)

* * *

The sweet snack choices in the 600 calorie breakfast prompted *Science Daily* to title its piece, "New Diet: Top Off Breakfast With—Chocolate Cake?" That sensationalized the solid and useful content of the study. I believe it clouded the key point of the Israeli study, which is simply that a hearty balanced breakfast puts you in the frame of mind to eat sensibly for the rest of the day. A low-carb, low-calorie breakfast, on the other hand, puts food uppermost in your mind for the rest of the day; self control holds up for a few days or even weeks, but you eventually—inevitably—give in.

It was not necessary to include dessert choices in the Jakubowicz study. Feelings of hunger and deprivation could have been avoided by filling out the 600 calorie breakfast with fruit, nuts, skim milk, whole grains, and perhaps a little sugar or artificial sweetener. An egg or a small fish fillet would've also been good choices, adding protein and good fat. I believe the results would've been the same, perhaps better, in the long run. Those changes would've allowed the participants to eat more volume, chew more, and feel more satisfied. Needless to say, it would've also served them better nutritionally.

That's what I have for breakfast. I leave the table feeling satisfied—and I don't crave sweets. The cravings in the Jakubowicz study came from lack of calories and carbohydrates—not lack of sweets.

If I don't have sweets, I don't crave sweets. But once I have the first bite, I'm off and running. One piece of chocolate cake with breakfast would leave me wanting another piece later in the day. Maybe that's just me, but I don't think so.

The key is to keep sweets out of sight and out of mind. As long as I can't see, smell, or taste sweets, I'm perfectly fine. I believe most people are the same. (This doesn't mean I don't have a sweet treat occasionally.)

It is true, of course, that hunger and deprivation must be avoided. That is the secret of long term weight control. The Israeli researchers proved that brilliantly. They just went a little overboard.

(Most active men and women would also require more total

calories to feel full and satisfied; 1600 calories would not be enough for me.)

* * *

In dieting, as we've seen, we often defeat ourselves by attempting to override our nature. That doesn't work; it's bad physiology. It's also bad psychology, weakening our will and destroying our motivation.

Let's dig deeper and look at the impact of personality and attitude on fitness, health, and longevity.

Chapter Eleven
Personality Traits

The Longevity Project

"It's not the happy-go-lucky who thrive—it's the prudent and persistent who flourish through the years," psychologists Howard S. Friedman, PhD, and Leslie R. Martin, PhD, wrote in *The Longevity Project* (Hudson Street, 2011).

The Longevity Project reveals that personality traits, relationships, experiences, and career paths have an effect on our health and longevity—often in surprising ways. Fortunately, many life enhancing personality traits can be cultivated. We can do far more for ourselves than others can do for us. We are the vanguard of our health.

Friedman and Martin used one of the most celebrated studies in psychology to answer the question of who lives longest—and why. They used a study of 1500 precocious children begun in 1921 by Stanford University psychologist Lewis Terman and carried on by others into this century. The beauty of the study, what makes it unique, is that the children were studied in meticulous detail throughout the course of their lives. Almost all of them are now gone. So we know how they lived, when they died, and what caused their death. Some died early and others had long and healthy lives.

Dr. Terman's study, begun 90 years ago, has become a veritable gold mine of information for several generations of researchers. Friedman and Martin began mining and contributing to the Terman study in 1990, an auspicious time when the children were in their ninth decade of life or deceased. Their findings are chronicled in *The Longevity Project.*

"The patterns and pathways to long life that we have uncovered make a significant difference in health and longevity—on average, many account for five or more years of life," the authors wrote. "If you put them together, you find the reasons why many bright, healthy children live to their seventies, eighties, and even nineties or hundreds, while many other bright, healthy children go on to die in their fifties and sixties."

The best childhood predictor of longevity was conscientiousness—the qualities of a prudent, persistent, well-organized person—somewhat obsessive and not at all carefree. That may not be sexy and exciting but, as we'll see, it's quite logical.

Some might have predicted that cheerfulness or a sociable personality would be the best predictor of a long life, but that was clearly not the case. "Certain other factors were also relevant, but the prudent, dependable children lived longest," the authors state without equivocation. "The strength of this finding was unexpected, but it proved to be a very important and enduring one."

To confirm his earlier evaluations Dr. Terman gave his subjects a new series of tests and measures of conscientiousness in 1940, when they were adults. Friedman and Martin also tested Terman's questions and measures on contemporary subjects, and compared the results using modern, well validated personality tests.

Dr. Terman's approach to personality holds up nicely and can help predict our own futures. "This confirmation in adulthood was particularly impressive because personality was being measured differently," the authors explained. Conscientiousness in childhood was measured by parent and teacher ratings. Conscientiousness in adulthood was measured by self-report questionnaires.

Finally, Friedman and Martin did something earlier researchers could not have done. They matched conscientiousness ratings with death certificates. By the end of the twentieth century, 70 percent of the Terman men and 51 percent of the Terman women had died. "It was the unconscientious among them who had been dying in especially large numbers," the authors wrote. "In both cases—childhood and adulthood—conscientiousness was the key personality predictor of long life."

Why is conscientiousness so important? The authors give three possible reasons why conscientious individuals tend to stay healthier and live longer. "To our great surprise, all three are true," they wrote.

The first reason is perhaps the most obvious. "Conscientious people do more things to protect their health and engage in fewer activities that are risky," the authors reported. They are less likely to smoke or drive too fast, for example. They buckle their seat belt and follow the doctor's advice. "They are not necessarily risk averse but they tend to be sensible in evaluating how far to push the envelope."

Second, and least obvious, some people are biologically predisposed to be both more conscientious and healthier. They're less prone to develop certain diseases, and not just those caused by dangerous habits. "We and others are uncovering this startling finding again and again—conscientious folks are less likely to die from all sorts of causes," the authors wrote. "While we are not yet sure of the precise physiological reasons, it appears that conscientious and unconscientious people have different levels of certain chemicals in their brains, including serotonin... Individuals with low levels of serotonin tend to be much more impulsive. Importantly, serotonin is also necessary to regulate many health-related processes throughout the body, including how much you eat and how well you sleep."

Fortunately, there is no cause for fatalism. Levels of neurotransmitters such as serotonin can change over time. Some Terman subjects who started out low on conscientiousness led long and healthy lives. "Some wild frat boys quit drinking the morning after their fortieth birthday," the authors reassured readers. "Cautious others abandon their sensible lifestyle in midlife and buy a red sports convertible."

The third and final reason is perhaps the most hopeful and empowering. Having a conscientious personality can lead you into healthier situations and relationships. "[Conscientious people] find their way to happier marriages, better friendships, and healthier work situations," the authors wrote. "That's right, conscientious people create healthy, long-life pathways for themselves."

* * *

My favorite portion of the book was *Jocks versus Nerds*. The Terman study, of course, started well before fitness was cool. Jack LaLanne was six years old when Dr. Terman picked his first subject. It was more than four decades before Dr. Ken Cooper coined the term *aerobics*. P90X and CrossFit were beyond the imagination of the most farsighted Termanator. Nevertheless, the Terman study participants have an important message for us on staying physically active throughout life.

Friedman and Martin began with a personal example.

Co-author Leslie Martin climbed Mt. Kilimanjaro in 2005, and recently completed the 151-mile Marathon des Sables across the Moroccan Sahara. The 6-day Marathon des Sables crosses the hottest part of Africa; runners have to carry their own food, bedding, and clothing the whole way. She enjoys the challenge of extreme sports, but for personal fulfillment as part of her active lifestyle—not for health reasons. Ultradistance events suit her, but she doesn't urge that lifestyle on others. She recommends whatever "gets you up and out of your chair."

That's essentially what active, healthy Terman participants did.

"Fitness levels, it appears, are more personal than the general *exercise is good for you* mantra might suggest," Friedman and Martin wrote. "All in all the findings told us that it makes no sense to rely on generalizations—individuals, we found, are on their own activity paths. The edict to exercise rigorously needs to be altered and tailored to the person."

"If you don't like jogging, don't jog," the authors advised. "Instead, begin doing things that you really enjoy and can keep up... You don't have to do the same thing all the time, and you definitely don't have to do something that irritates or bores you."

Nerds in childhood often won out in the long run. Being a childhood jock did not lead to long life if you were one of those who quit sports and slowed down a lot as you aged. On the other hand, being inactive in childhood was not a problem if you became more active as you aged. "Those who were active in youth and stayed active tended to live very long lives," the authors reported. "Those who were inactive in youth and became more active often did almost as well in terms of life span, and sometimes equally well."

Find an activity or activities that suit your personality. Mark Twain found exercise loathsome, but the authors say he had the right idea generally. His maxim: "We can't reach old age by another man's road. My habits protect my life, but they would assassinate you."

* * *

We'll end with a look at extroverts, outgoing and gregarious, and introverts, shy and reclusive. Which personality type is most likely to have a long and healthy life? Many will find the topic revealing and perhaps encouraging, as I did.

The surprising news here is that sociability isn't as health protective as one might think. "Being a 'people person' can have its benefits, but those who rank high on sociability often find themselves in environments that encourage unhealthy behaviors—and they join in the dangers of the moment," the authors related.

It pays to be selective in your socializing, according to Friedman and Martin. Friendly people who choose wisely reaped long term health benefits. Many of the more introverted children grew up to take on stable jobs and develop steady friendships, which were just as valuable for health and long life. "So if you're socially reluctant and you're okay with that—so are we."

Friedman and Martin found that, on average, sociable children did not live longer. Some died young, while others lived into old age. It was roughly a wash. It does, of course, make a difference whether a person is friendly and outgoing or someone who works well alone and doesn't much care for parties. For example, people high on the sociability scale are usually excellent in sales. On the other hand, introverts often do better in science or research fields.

One of Dr. Terman's last studies, in 1954, posed the question *Are scientists different?* He was wondering how to recruit more scholars to be scientists and also how to smooth relations between scientists and lawyers. What he found revealed a lot about the gulf between extroverts and introverts.

Terman concluded that scientists and engineers are at the opposite pole from businessmen and lawyers in their abilities, occupational interests, and social behaviors. Scientists were much less sociable. In school, future scientists were shyer and less involved in social networks.

"These differences were just what we needed—an important clue as to why sociability did not predict who lived a long life," the authors wrote.

After recreating Terman's groups of scientists and nonscientists, Friedman and Martin found that scientists outlived the nonscientists. "Only two-thirds of the nonscientists but almost three-quarters of the scientists lived to reach age seventy."

Importantly, the two groups were equal in conscientiousness. So why didn't the sociable lawyers and businessmen live longer?

"It turns out the scientists had an ace in the whole," the authors explained. "They tended to move into stable jobs, have long-lasting marriages, and generally work in a responsible manner. Nonscientists—that is, the businessmen, lawyers, salesman, and so on—tended to have more tumultuous, less stable, and more health-damaging careers and behaviors."

"Overall, [however], sociability was a wash. It didn't help or harm one's expected life span."

* * *

The lesson, it seems to me, is that it would pay to think long and hard about where you fall on the personality scale before you choose or change a career—or fitness—path. It may explain why I have found more satisfaction in studying and writing about health and fitness than I did in practicing law. On the other hand, the ability to think clearly and logically, as required for success in law school and law practice, has been extremely helpful to my career as a fitness writer and consultant. So it may be that I chose more wisely than I knew, at the beginning and at the turning point.

Personality may also explain why training alone in our gym works for me, when others do better with the comradery provided by a commercial gym or fitness center. Conscientiousness helps either way.

Conscientiousness pays off in the gym, at work, and in life.

* * *

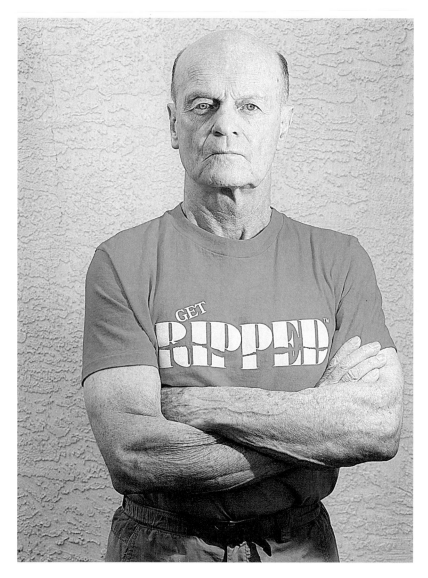

While my personality may not have been a good fit for law, law school and practice were excellent preparation for studying and writing about health and fitness. *Photo by Laszlo Bencze*

With that background, let's look at the role of attitude, optimism and pessimism, in the fitness and health equation.

Attitude Matters

I've long believed in the power of positive thinking. We are far more likely to succeed if we expect to succeed. We can do amazing things with the right attitude.

John North, who died at 85 (while this book was being written) from the same cancer that took his father at 62, was one of the most positive people I've ever known. He told me a story some years ago that reflected his approach to life. He and his stepson Gary had just finished rebuilding the engine on a 1985 Buick. I'll use his words—he delighted in writing carefully crafted letters detailing important principles:

We both have worked on engines before, but neither of us had tackled one of the new computer-controlled front-wheel-drive engines before. When we opened the hood, it looked like a plate of spaghetti—there were so many wires, hoses and assorted thingamajigs. Most people would have thought it was hopeless. But we piled right in.

It took us four days to assemble and install the new parts. The last hurdle was reprogramming the onboard computer.

The engine started right up. With a few adjustments we had it running like new.

How many people would have said, "No way!" Gary and I don't think that way. The truth is, we can do almost anything if we believe we can.

John had a valid point. *In Learned Optimism* (Alfred A. Knopf, 1991) Martin E. P. Seligman, PhD, one of the world's leading authorities on motivation, presented scientific evidence that optimists get along better than pessimists in almost every facet of life: school, work, personal relationships, sports—you name it. According to Seligman, optimists respond better to adversity of all kinds. What's more, they have better physical health and may even live longer. The key seems to be what we say to ourselves when we confront failure and disappointment.

Pessimists, according to Seligman, respond with helplessness; they give up. Optimists, on the other hand, persevere. Like John and Gary, they assess the situation, and they act constructively. Importantly, our "explanatory style"—Seligman's term for the manner in which we explain setbacks to ourselves—can

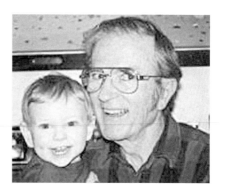

This is our favorite photo of John, taken in 1997 with his step-grandson. It's how we'll always remember him.
Photo by John North

even affect our immune system; optimists tend to have better immune activity than pessimists.

Most of us learn to be optimists or pessimists in childhood and adolescence, and then, for good or bad, we carry this basic attitude with us throughout life. Nevertheless, a negative explanatory cycle can be changed to positive.

The pioneering research done by Seligman and his colleagues on learned helplessness or optimism is a revelation.

In 1965, Seligman, while a graduate student in the department of experimental psychology at the University of Pennsylvania, performed the first experiment showing that animals can be taught helplessness. One group of dogs was given escapable shock. By pushing a panel with its nose, a dog in that group could turn off the shock. A second group of dogs was given exactly the same shocks as the first, but no response they made had any effect. They had no control; they couldn't escape. A third group was given no shocks at all.

Once the dogs went through the experiment, each was put in a large box with two compartments, separated by a low wall. In the first compartment they received a shock, but they could easily escape the shock by jumping over the barrier into the other side of the box.

Within seconds the dogs that had been taught to control shocks discovered that they could jump over the barrier and escape. The dogs that earlier had received no shocks discovered the same thing, also in a matter of seconds. But the dogs who had found that nothing they did mattered made no effort to escape, even though they could easily see over the low barrier to the shock-less zone of the box.

Those dogs just gave up and lay down, even though they were being regularly shocked by the box. They never found that they could easily escape. Those dogs had learned that they had no control, that they were helpless.

It turned out that learned helplessness has far-reaching effects. In 1977, Madelon Visintainer, one of Seligman's graduate students, performed an experiment showing how mastery and helplessness can affect health. She put three groups of rats through the same shock experiment as Seligman had with the dogs, but with an important addition. The day before the experiment she implanted a few cancer cells on each rat's flank.

Under normal conditions, 50% of the rats would reject the cancer cells and live. As expected, 50% of the rats who were not shocked had died, and the other half had rejected the tumor. Of the rats who were allowed to escape the shock by pressing a bar, the rats that had learned mastery, 70% rejected the tumor. But only 27% of the helpless rats, the rats who had experienced uncontrollable shock, rejected the cancer cells. In short, Visintainer became the first person to demonstrate that the psychological state of helplessness produces a more rapid growth of cancer. She also showed, of course, that the psychological state of mastery enhances the ability to reject the tumor. And that's not all. Visintainer went on to demonstrate that the rats that had experienced mastery when young were better protected against tumors as adults.

Seligman said it works the same way in humans. Researchers at Yale found that elderly people in nursing homes were not only happier when they were given greater control over the daily happenings in their lives, but they also lived longer.

Optimists have also been found to have better immune activity than pessimists. For example, Seligman and his colleagues taught learned optimism to 40 cancer patients and produced a very sharp increase in the activity of natural killer cells, the cells that kill foreign invaders in the body, such as viruses, bacteria, and tumor cells.

Perhaps that explains why John North was able to sidestep the lethal cancer for 23 years longer than his father.

* * *

While I haven't had to deal with anything as serious as cancer, weight training has had a powerful influence on my life. I started lifting weights at about 13, and I believe it gave me a positive outlook on life, an optimistic frame of reference that has stayed with me throughout my life.

Weight training taught me that what I did counted, that I had the power to shape the course of my life. I was small for my age and I think I felt a little inferior. I wanted to change that, and I did. I wanted to be as strong as—no, stronger than—my school buddies. Through weight training, I not only matched my athletic friends, I surpassed them. As a junior I won the state high school pentathlon championship, a five-event contest consisting of push-ups, chin-ups, jump reach, bar vault, and 300-yard shuttle run. Over the next decade or so, I became a city, state, and regional champion in Olympic weightlifting.

Weight training taught me that if I set realistic goals and worked hard and intelligently, I would succeed. Those early successes taught me that perseverance pays. They set the pattern for the rest of my life, a pattern which has extended far beyond sports. For instance, the stick-to-itiveness that I learned through weight training helped me graduate second in my class from a law school that flunked four out of five entering students. It has helped me in everything I've attempted since then.

I am also convinced that positive thinking, combined with constructive action, has given me exceptional health.

*　*　*

Fast forward to the April 17, 2012, issue of *Psychological Bulletin*, where researchers from the Harvard School of Public Health published findings that positive psychological well-being appears to reduce the risk of heart attacks, strokes, and other cardiovascular events. In short, an optimistic outlook on life fosters good health.

We've long believed that negative mental states, such as depression, anger, anxiety, and hostility, are harmful to cardiovascular health. A systematic review of more than 200 studies by research fellow Julia K. Boehm and associate professor Laura D. Kubzansky found that the reverse is also true. A positive mental state appears to promote good health. Boehm and Kubzansky found the association between optimism and heart health to be especially noteworthy.

"We found that factors such as optimism, life satisfaction, and happiness are associated with reduced risk of cardiovascular diseases...," said Boehm. "For example, the most optimistic individuals had an approximately 50% reduced risk of experiencing an initial cardiovascular event, compared to their less optimistic peers."

As with most findings of this kind, it's not as simple as it sounds. "The absence of the negative is not the same as the presence of the positive," Boehm cautioned.

People with a positive sense of well-being tend to have healthier blood pressure, cholesterol, and weight, and are also more likely to exercise, eat healthy, get enough sleep, and avoid smoking. So we have a chicken or egg issue. We don't know whether a positive outlook makes people more inclined to take care of themselves—or whether healthy living makes people feel more optimistic. Boehm says it will take more research to tease out whether the positive outlook or the heart-healthy behavior comes first.

It makes little practical difference. We win either way. If a positive outlook makes us more inclined to exercise and eat healthy, we win. But we also win if exercise and healthy eating make us happy and motivates us to stay the course.

It works for me either way. My dad motivated me to start training with weights. Once I saw the positive results, wild horses couldn't have stopped me. Dr. Seligman would call that learned optimism.

Chapter Twelve

Take Charge People

My father was the quintessential *Take Charge* person; he did things the way that worked best for him. It was a family trait. His father and grandfather were the same way. No one told them what to do or how to think; they decided on a course of action and stuck to it as long as it was working. They were strong willed—and successful—men. All three were medical doctors.

My paternal grandfather and namesake perhaps summed it up best: "A man convinced against his will is of the same opinion still."

The family mindset was in play early for my dad. He came home in the first grade with a report that he was misbehaving and failing. His father told him in no uncertain terms that that was unacceptable; he put the fear of God in him. I never had the opportunity to ask my grandfather about it; he was killed in a car accident the year before I was born. I was told that he threatened to beat my dad within an inch of his life if he didn't shape up. Whatever the message, it got through loud and clear. My dad got straight-As from that point forward, all the way through medical school. In medical school if you got an A in all the exams during the term, you didn't have to take the final exam. He never had to take a final exam.

My father excelled in just about everything he put his mind to, including athletics.

He grew up in a time when exercise wasn't the "in" thing, and he was always busy practicing medicine. He did things he enjoyed—ping pong, punching the bag, chin-ups—from time to time, but nothing regular. He didn't walk, run, or lift weights.

But he was a track and field star in his youth, excelling in the discus, broad jump, high jump, and pole vault.

He placed third in the New Mexico High School Track and Field Championship—as a team. He was the whole team. That's hard to believe, I know, but I received confirmation this past year from Terry Gent, a sports historian doing research on the occasion of the 100-year anniversary of our state meet; New Mexico became a state in 1912. It turns out that the story is even better than I'd been led to believe.

Mr. Gent sent me some heart warming—and absolutely priceless—newspaper clippings from the *Albuquerque Morning Journal* on my dad's exploits.

The Saturday, May 14, 1921, edition reported on my dad's first appearance in the state meet: "Bass of Cimarron, a youngster of about 15 years, appeared on the field [in the prelims] in his everyday clothes, and placed in the high jump, clearing the bar against his older opponents who had the usual advantage of a track suit. Arrangements were made to get the lad a track suit today and he will bear watching in this event."

Here's what happened later on that day in the finals, Gent related: "Your dad won and jumped 5 feet 7 inches, which was ¾ of an inch below the state record. He was 14 or 15 years old; I still can't determine. Regardless, he was the youngest State Champ at that time." (The Sunday paper confirmed that he was 14.)

Gent said a few boys of 14 years have won state titles in the 100 years of the state meet—"But very few." There was no age limit at that time, so he was competing against many 19- and 20-year-olds. "And possibly some 21."

"In 1922, your father tied for the high jump title with Orville Zillmer [of] Albuquerque High School." Gent wrote in a follow-up letter. "He was 15 years old while Orville was 21," he added. My dad's last appearance in the State Meet was in 1923. (He finished high school—and the first two years of college—at the New Mexico Military Institute in Roswell, which didn't participate in the state meet.) "He was the 'High Point Man' in 1923, at 16!! And placed 3rd in the team competition, alone," Mr. Gent confirmed. So it's true and— because of his age—even more remarkable than I knew.

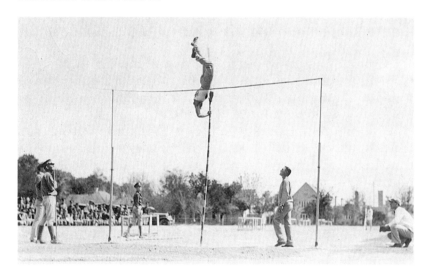

This photo, taken at the New Mexico Military Institute in 1926, shows my dad pole-vaulting; he came within an inch or two of the world record. "Your dad, most likely, used a hardwood pole throughout his career and had to land on his feet at ground level in a dirt pit," Mr. Gent wrote. *Photographer unknown*

The 1926 N.M.M.I. yearbook said of my dad: "For sportsman-ship, pole-vaulting, soldiering, and hard-headedness" he was supreme. That tells you a lot about the kind of man he was.

After that, he went from one success to another, in medicine and real estate development. He practiced medicine for about 50 years—including a few years in the Army Air Force during WW II—and was loved and respected by his patients. He had a taste for fast cars—in his boyhood there was over 100 makes of automobiles and he could tell you about every one of them—and over the years owned some of the best ones. We have photos of some of his most memorable cars in our home.

My dad lived life on his own terms. Hard-headed? Yes. He did things his way; that's for sure. He was a good man and, follow-ing in the footsteps of his father, a wonderful father. He encour-aged me always, but never pushed me to do anything against my will. Gone for 26 years, he still gives me strength.

I'd also like to tell you about five of my *Take Charge* friends, all successful in their own way, each story different. As I've written before, "Surely the quickest path to disillusionment is the one blazed by someone else." We can benefit from their examples, not by emulating them, but by appreciating their uniqueness and drawing inspiration to find our own way.

Truck Driver on the Road to Fitness

Carol and I met Steve Schultz as he was passing through Al-buquerque. He called ahead; saying he'd read our books and would like to meet us. Wondering what we might be getting our-selves into, we agreed. It was the right decision.

We spent a delightful 90 minutes or so talking with him at a truck stop a few miles west of town. We'd never really taken a close look at a large truck stop; it was fascinating with perhaps 50 rigs lined up in military-like precision, with all the neces-sary amenities at hand. He showed us the high-tech gauges and controls in the cockpit of his state-of-the-art truck—we had no idea it was so complex—and over lunch he regaled us with his well thought-out plan for eating wisely and working out on the road.

Impressed, we asked him to spell it out in more detail for our readers. His amazing story generated interest like nothing else of its kind posted on our website. Once plausible excuses for missed workouts and fast food on the run were vaporized.

This is what he wrote:

I am an over-the-road, cross-country truck driver. Forty-nine years old and sitting behind the wheel of an eighteen wheeler for nine to 10 hours a day, and being away from home 10 to 12 days at a time, you can imagine that a horrible cycle of inactivity and poor food choices could make me unfit, unhealthy, and fat. The majority of truck drivers are just that, overweight, inactive, and suffering from myriad ailments.

Not only are we sitting most of the day, truck stop food is mostly buffet style and truckers are notorious for eating only once or twice a day because of scheduled deliveries. Eating proper portions does not enter into the average driver's mind when he does get to finally sit down and eat a meal. Being away from home and family, comfort food is on your mind, and lots of it.

Be that as it may, I have found my way to a very fit lifestyle by using the principles in Clarence's books—and my own ingenuity.

I eat four small meals a day and find a way to exercise almost every day. I drive a Peterbilt with a sleeper behind the cab. There is plenty of room for two electric coolers and a microwave oven. I can pull into any rest area, prepare and eat a healthy meal in 30 minutes. Here is what I eat every day (Clarence's uniform eating plan).

Breakfast *is my version of Clarence's "Old Reliable:"*

> *Half cup cooked grains (I precook grains at home: oat groats, barely, rye, buckwheat and kamut)*
> *Half cup light vanilla soy milk*
> *One chopped apple*
> *Tablespoon chopped walnuts*

Meal 2:

> *One hardboiled egg (split) between two whole wheat tortillas (50 cal each), along with chopped peppers and onions, mustard, grape tomatoes, and bean sprouts*
> *For dessert, I have .5 cup of fat free cottage cheese with .5 cup of chopped cantaloupe or honeydew and a heaping tbs. of ground flax seed*

Meal 3:

> *A whole wheat pita (60 cal) with hummus, black beans (home cooked, no salt), Pico de Gallo, broccoli slaw, and hot sauce*
> *Dessert: same as meal 2*

Meal 4: *(I alternate between three different dinners)*

> *1. Half-cup egg beaters, onions and peppers, yellow squash and zucchini, plus three corn tortillas (I have found a brand that has only 25 calories each)*
> *2. Pizza, consisting of two whole wheat tortillas, pizza sauce,*

197

onions and peppers, squash and zucchini, pineapple chunks, low fat mozzarella cheese, and a few chopped black olives

3. Stir fry veggie mix, tofu, pineapple chunks, 1-2 tbs. Thai sauce (low sodium) served on a bed of Quinoa (.5 cup)

Dessert: 3/4 cup of plain fat free yogurt, with a .5 cup mixed berries, and ground flax seed

I am never hungry on this whole-food diet, but it's quite a scene at home the day before I leave on my next trip. My wife and I are chopping peppers and onions, cutting up melon, cooking grain, boiling the eggs. Preparation is half the battle.

Truck stops can also be a road block to exercise; they are quite often situated outside of large cities, along highways where walking or running is prohibited or unsafe.

I carry a couple of adjustable dumbbells, which permit me to do a complete lifting routine. I have also found wonderful and inspiring places along my travels for hiking or running. For example:

The rest area on top of Donner Pass in California's Sierra Nevada Mountains is great place for a high altitude hike—wonderful for your attitude.

I like to run on a stretch of old route 66 in Arizona that runs parallel to Meteor Crater.

I have also climbed rock piles in west Texas and Wyoming, and hiked the Appalachian Trail in Pennsylvania.

I make my home in a small town where everyone knows everyone. It's a very friendly place to live and raise a family. When I'm home, I love to walk around and checkout the parks or visit Main Street.

As you can see, I get around and try to make the best of every situation. I have even found myself under the trailer on a rainy day doing push ups and prone pull-ups.

I started on this road to fitness in 2002 when I felt myself living a little too loosely, as in too little exercise and a lot of poor eating habits. With two of my children entering their teens, I decided it was time to set a good example.

I pulled out some back issues of Muscle and Fitness and re-read some of Clarence's columns from the early nineties. I then found his website and ordered some of his books, which often contain excerpts from other great books.

One in particular was Dr. Ken Cooper's classic Aerobics. I started running and found that I enjoyed it. Cooper's book has a fitness test where you see how far you can run in 12 minutes. I persuaded my son and daughter to try it with me; they both *did poorly, while old dad was in the good category. They would have none of that, and kept at it until they passed the test and then some. They both joined the track and cross country teams in high school and have excelled. My daughter Stephanie is now a three sport college athlete and Tyler made the varsity squad as a freshman. With my youngest, Teague, nine, now lifting weights with me—it's one of his favorite activities—Clarence's inspiration has reached two generations in my family so far.*

I have been at this type of lifestyle for five years and counting. I am 5-10, 165 pounds, with a fairly low body fat %. I make my home in SW Minnesota.

* * *

Where there's a will, there's a way. Steve Schultz is a wonderful example.

Checking in with Steve before writing this, we learned that his story has another part, one that is both unfortunate and uplifting. Steve and his wife have divorced. We are not privy to the details, but we do know that Steve is still on the road to fitness. Again, we'll let him tell you about it:

In 2009, I became single.

I soon met a wonderful woman from South Dakota who was active and health conscious like me. She was a traveling nurse and we saw each other sporadically. Then in November 2010 we decided to locate in Sioux Falls with jobs that allowed us to have a more traditional lifestyle.

I now pull a tanker with liquid eggs from a farm in Nebraska to a production facility in Minnesota. I pack my lunch with the same healthy foods I ate while driving over the road. My girlfriend can't figure out how I can eat the same thing everyday, but I keep telling her that it's good fresh food, and I know it's doing me good so the enjoyment comes from more than just taste.

Now everything wasn't all that cheery after the dissolution of my marriage; it isn't a pleasant experience. Moving to a new city and with a new job routine, my diet suffered as did my exercise habits.

With all the big changes to my life I found myself eating out more often and letting my workouts slide. Less activity meant weight gain and that set me up for feelings of lethargy which, in the nasty cycle of things, lead to more weight gain.

My running seemed difficult and I did less and less of it; weight training was a chore.

It took my new girlfriend's desire to learn about eating right, staying fit and keeping healthy to get myself motivated and put my health goals back on track. I've learned that you must be ever vigilant; it is so easy to slide into an unhealthy lifestyle.

So with that we dialed in our calories with the use of an app on our smart phones to track daily calorie intake and the amount of calories burned during exercise. We get excellent feedback, and it really helps.

Although I eat a vegetarian diet, Sylvia eats more like Clarence's flexitarian style with grass fed beef from her father's farm and chicken that her mother raises as side dishes. I like the volumetrics style of eating while she needs to work on fitting a few more high-calorie foods into her hectic ER routine.

I lift two to three times a week, incorporating a push and a pull movement along with squats or deadlifts. We bike, run, or walk on the other days. When we have time off you can find us biking or hiking. We've been kayaking this summer and we recently climbed Harney's Peak in the Black Hills and explored the Badlands of western South Dakota. We also went white water

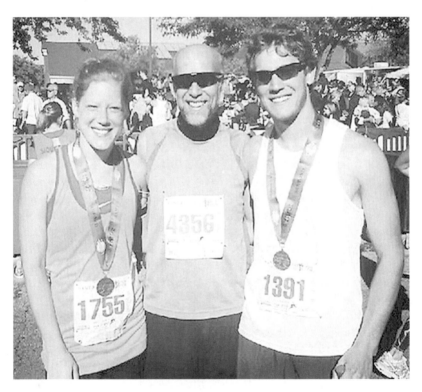

Steve and his children continue to share an active lifestyle. Here you see him with his daughter Stephanie and son Tyler at the 2012 Sioux Falls marathon. *Steve provided us with this photo.*

rafting on the Colorado River and hiking the Grand Mesa in Colorado. Keeping active can be so much fun!

* * *

Life changes bring with them new challenges. People like Steve Schultz roll with the punches and find a way to stay on the road to fitness.

Businessman Rises to Fitness Challenge

Martin (not his real name) wrote to me about three years ago. We were not to meet until some time later, but his letter stood out in my memory. Clearly this man was special, a rare breed.

After climbing to the top of the corporate world, he retired at an early age to pursue private investing, charitable and other interests. Unfortunately, things didn't go as he had hoped. Several years into retirement he encountered a serious health problem. His blood pressure rose alarmingly. Testing revealed a cancerous mass in a vital organ. Surgery successfully removed the cancer, but left him vulnerable to other complications.

Martin discovered me years ago in *Muscle & Fitness* magazine and had read my books. "You have been an inspiration to me for thirty years," he wrote. He had been training and watching his diet for many years. He achieved a very low body fat and a fitness level rarely seen in hard charging businessmen. This allowed him to work longer hours and move ahead faster than his contemporaries. "I benefited in my work substantially from a greater sense of well being and more stamina," he wrote in his letter.

He trained vigorously in the period leading up to his cancer surgery, but began to slack off in his training and diet afterward. Something happened after the surgery. "I no longer was as diligent about going to the gym...and stopped being disciplined in my eating," he wrote. For the first time he lost the drive to train and eat healthy. His encounter with mortality appeared to sap his desire to stay fit.

Predictably, he put on weight. In a few short years, he saw his body fat rise to 25%. He no longer stood out from his age-group peers; he joined the crowd. But he didn't stay there for long.

"Over the last year, I have reduced my weight to 175, and my body fat to 18%, and stopped taking all medication," he wrote near the end of his letter. Best of all, he planned to slowly reduce his body fat over the next year and be back to 165 and 11% fat, where he was before his cancer scare.

"My life is improved from reading about yours," he wrote in closing.

When I next heard from him a year later he had lost the additional 10 pounds, achieved his 165 target weight—but there was a problem. He lacked motivation; he was spinning his wheels, making no progress.

"I used to (30 years ago) really look forward to weight training, but have lost that enthusiasm and would like to regain it," he told me. "My goal has become to get through the workout!"

I suggested that he spend a few days eating and training with us in Albuquerque. A few weeks later he flew in on a chartered flight. We had a wonderful time talking, eating, and training together. He was a sponge, eagerly soaking up everything that was said or done.

I told him that I have goals for every workout. I explained that I sit down with my training diary before every workout. I showed him how I review what I did the last time. I rotate through a number of different workouts, so the last time for that workout is usually two weeks back; it would be almost impossible to keep track without a training diary of some kind. My diary allows me to set specific goals for each workout. Goal setting is an art. The key is to be realistic—and set yourself up for success. (I rarely fail to improve in some way.) That makes every workout an exciting and rewarding experience.

Martin was quick to see the value in that approach. So simple and yet so powerful!

We did ten 250-meter intervals on the Concept 2 rower. I showed him my pace on each rep in the last workout, and then did slightly better on nine out of 10 reps. He took to it right away. The next time I heard from him he was making steady progress. His rowing times were improving by leaps and bounds.

Rapport was excellent during Martin's visit; we discussed many diet and training issues and had a marvelous exchange. He said his time with us was some of the most productive of his life.

It was a wonderful compliment, but I don't let it go to my head. The point is that he didn't have to shower me with praise. It's what successful people do; they give credit for performance. Recognize performance and you're likely to get more of it. Praise doesn't cost anything; it pays to give it generously.

Martin is motivated and willing to learn. When he has problems—with exercise, health, or whatever—he reaches out and finds a solution.

Every time we hear from him he has an exciting new fitness goal. He took my idea—challenge brings success—and made it his own. That's what *Take Charge* people do.

Deborah Finds Her Way

Deborah Nyberg is a determined lady from Norway; she knows her mind and her body. Not willing to settle for the ordinary, she wants a fitness regimen that suits her—and she's willing to keep looking until she finds it. She's also flexible; when one diet or exercise plan stops working for her, she looks for something else. When her circumstances change, she adjusts. She is relentless in her pursuit of fitness.

Her twists and turns over the years are a case study in thoughtful—and purposeful—training.

I encourage people to think for themselves—and she does.

This is her story in her own words:

The first time I saw Clarence Bass was on the front cover of Challenge Yourself. *My husband had bought the book and thought it might interest me since I was looking for ways of making our diet healthier and restart my training routine. I remember being amazed at the way Bass looked at age 60. How could this be? Well, the truth seemed to be much simpler than I had expected. There were no gimmicks, no funky diet techniques, just common sense.*

That was ten years ago. Although my road to fat loss and fitness has had its ups and downs, Clarence has been there all the way through his books (my husband bought all nine), encouraging me to do what feels right.

Clarence is adamant about the ownership principle—read, learn, and adapt. Read the details of his journey, learn the lessons, and then adapt the parts that make sense to you into your lifestyle, one step at a time.

I've never been one to follow in someone else's footsteps. The combination of Clarence's sound advice and what I feel is right for me has carried me through a wonderful journey. What is remarkable is that each time I stray—and I do—Clarence's books are always there to guide me back onto my path.

Years ago, I thought I wanted to be a body builder and did weight lifting for about 3 years, with very good gains, but finally came to realize that my total enjoyment lies in activities that require a combination of strength and endurance. I engaged in a variety of physical activities, hoping to find one that fit into the strength and endurance category, while providing a promising future based on my true abilities.

At the end of October 2008, I rediscovered indoor rowing (we have owned a Concept 2 Rower for a few years) and felt like a spark had been ignited. Again, Clarence Bass was an inspiration. He is an avid Concept 2 rower. The 5000 meter row was the first competitive distance I tried, landing me [in 29th place] on the Concept 2 World Ranking List (Lightweight Women, 30-39). After a few months of rowing workouts (walking on off days), I've managed to progress to 12th place. I hope to be in the top ten in a couple of months. So it seems like I've found my sport.

On diet, I have also adopted the ownership principle. Whole grains for breakfast have never agreed with my digestion. My own "Old Reliable" is a delicious smoothie, made with kefir, banana, frozen berries and flax seeds. I do, however, use whole grains, fresh fruits and vegetables daily. My husband and I even invested in a grain mill a couple years ago, so that I could have fresh, whole spelt flour for my bread making.

Clarence Bass has taught me that you simply can't go wrong using fresh, whole foods. I have also found that consuming "good fats" in measured amounts agrees with my body.

I never tire of reading Clarence's books. I read them over and over again! I was very lucky to receive his latest book, Great Expectations *from my husband for my 37th birthday last year, along with two autographed pictures of Clarence. Those photos now hang in our office, over our Concept 2 rower. They are a constant reminder that aspiring for good health and fitness is an endless and worthwhile journey!*

My journey to good health and fitness will always have its ups and downs, but I've never given up and don't ever plan to. I'm happy to report that I am currently at my lowest weight since my early 20s and feel very fit and healthy.

I look forward to my workouts, knowing that I don't have to go all out; I can leave some effort for next time—another good tip from Clarence Bass' books (which he adapted from Bill Pearl), a tip which always improves my performance at my next workout. After years of procrastination, I finally summoned up the courage to write Clarence. I'm glad I did.

The mission statement on his website says: To inspire and help motivated people achieve lifelong leanness, health and total fitness

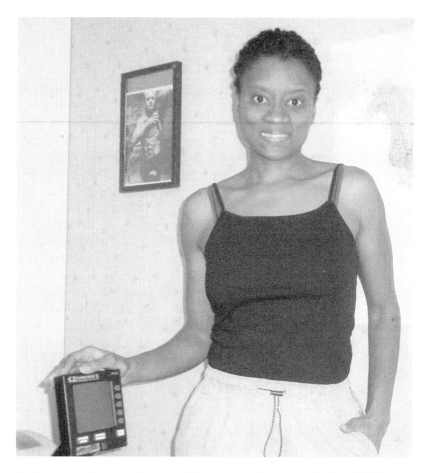

Deborah looking terrific—and 24 pounds lighter—with her C2 Rower, and our "Fab Ab" photo in the background.

Photo courtesy of Deborah Nyberg

Mission accomplished, Clarence and thank you!
Deborah Nyberg, Grimstad, Norway

[We next heard from Deborah a year later. Her training was still evolving and her progress continuing.]

I still have the same solid, common sense approach in place. This approach has accompanied me through over a decade of training and goes hand in hand with my way of thinking. It's a long-term approach you build on day after day, celebrating successes, large and small, along the way.

Weight: *I'm now about 2kg [4.4lbs] lighter than I was a year ago and one size smaller in clothes. A year ago, my fat percentage measured on my Tanita body composition scale was 24.6%*

(adult mode) or 19.6% (athletic mode). As of the 15th of May, this year, the readings are 22.1% / 17.6. In addition to losing fat, I have also gained a good amount of muscle. I would still like to lose a little more weight, but I've come to the point where even my hardest critic (me) has to admit that I look slender, with good muscle tone.

It's very motivating to look in the mirror and see a body that reflects my healthy lifestyle.

Meals: *My meals have varied slightly. For example, I now use soy milk in my breakfast smoothie, instead of kefir. I'm still consistently eating a healthy, whole food diet. I enjoy what I eat and look forward to each and every meal. I often fine tune what I eat, continually learning which foods work best for my body.*

Training: *I've had some good results during the 2010 rowing season and managed to set new PRs in all of my selected distances. The goal I set for myself last year, to be in the top ten on Concept 2's World Ranking for the 5000 meters, was accomplished. My official place for the 5000m at the end of the 2010 season was 8th out of 100 entrants. Out of my six distances in the 2010 season, I ended up in the top ten for five and in the top 25 for the hardest distance, the 2000m, which had a total of 116 entrants.*

[Moving up across six distances took effort and planning—a great example of using the performances of others to motivate yourself to do your best. You don't have to win, come first, to be a winner.]

The 2011 rowing season has just begun and I'm looking forward to new PRs in all of my distances.

I balance my rowing with off days to ensure adequate recovery. I do mostly walking on off days, but have done biking or running when the weather and my energy levels permit. I like the variation these other activities add to my training.

I've recently added Kettlebells to the strength aspect of my training and am already enjoying the challenge this new addition brings.

As Clarence said in his book Challenge Yourself, *setting goals is a major key to staying motivated. I thrive on the small successes. However, I've learned that challenges can't be undertaken at the cost of the long term goal, so I continue to value and respect rest days. If I'm too tired to give that extra bit, I usually don't. If a muscle doesn't feel right (for example I recently strained a back muscle indirectly through a non training incident) I back off for a while and lighten the training load. After all, my goal* is be active in training for the rest of my life, so knowing when to back off is as important as being brave enough to push hard when the time is right.

A friend of Bass mentioned that people should start "running" and never look back. I totally agree. Sometimes I've had to slow down, but I understand that the key is to keep going, while setting realistic goals along the way.

Like Clarence Bass, I have great expectations. I want to look good, feel great and challenge myself, year after year.

Thanks once again, Clarence, for giving me a lifetime of inspiration.

[Deborah wrote again, in April of 2012, with disturbing news.]

I've had a major life change within the past year. My husband and I are going through a separation. A very stressful process, but training, my belief in God, and support from family and friends are making sure that my girls and I get through this process with as little stress as possible.

My training habits changed after I moved into a new home with the girls. I found that I needed more down time to keep the stress levels down for me and the girls, so I stopped using the Concept 2 rower in the mornings, so that I could get extra sleep.

Since I am now working, I also stopping monitoring how long I walked and just made sure that I walked within the time I had, to and from work, to the grocery store, etc. The results have been very good. I have lost a little over 1 kg (I am now roughly 118 lbs), but have not lost my strength; in fact, I am still gaining strength. Family and friends have said that I look better than ever and I agree with them.

I now work out once a week: I do one hard Kettlebell session every Monday morning (I wake up at 0530, as I have done for the last couple of years) and that's it! The rest of the week is walking with a occasional bike ride, for pleasure only. I feel great and think I look better than I ever have. I'm happy with my progress.

My KB training is as follows:

Five sets of swings with a 44 lb bell. I have reached 35 reps for each set, so 5x35. (I plan to do 1 set of 40 reps and 4 sets of 35 tomorrow.) [A good choice, the KB swing strengthens the hips, back, and quads.]

I can also do 10 reps of the "Turkish Getup" with a 26 lb bell. The most I have done in a row is 7 with my left hand and 8 with my right. I am working on getting to 10 in a row. I do two other exercises as well and now use a range from 26lbs–44lbs for my Monday training session, which last just under an hour.

My eating habits are basically the same, with one exception. I no longer eat regular spelt bread; it happened accidentally, and I seem to be functioning better without it. I think I may have a problem with gluten. I am experimenting with gluten free bread. I still have my smoothie for breakfast every morning.

It's wonderful to be "there" and seen as a well trained woman. Even I have to admit, I've reached a certain level, a level I hoped to reach. I knew it was where I belonged, where I'm genetically suited to be.

It's wonderful to have people look at me in a way that I used to look at others, wondering what they do to keep their body in that shape or be simply amazed at their physique. I know some people feel I am "lucky," making the mistake of assuming I got where I am after a few weeks or months of hard work or following some crazy diet fad. I'm where I am due to my hard work, perseverance, belief in myself, my ability to adapt my training to the numerous changes in my lifestyle over the years, etc. One thing I know is that it's a great place to be and I'm not finished yet!

Warmest regards,
Deborah

Law Professor Thrives on Short, Efficient Workouts

While Dan Keating's doctorate is in law—he teaches bankruptcy and commercial law and has twice served as interim dean at Washington University School of Law in St. Louis—he knows his way around a gym like few others. He has the results to prove it.

Dan's heart is with muscle, but his body is more suited for endurance. He also has an amazing sense of coordination and balance. Wisely, he doesn't argue with success.

Among the tens of thousands tested at the Cooper Clinic in Dallas his treadmill time puts him in the top 1% for men his age. What's more, he can balance on one foot with his eyes closed almost indefinitely; if you don't think that's impressive, try it. Fifteen seconds is very good if you are 45 or older.

Those results—and more—were achieved with about two hours a week of training. He works out three times a week in his well-equipped basement. His workouts last about 40 minutes, 15 minutes weights and 25 aerobics.

Dan is a busy man; he works out in the morning before his

workday begins. His short, efficient workouts were born of necessity—and long experience. Not having much time for training, he has to make every minute count.

His weight workouts evolved over many years from the traditional volume approach into something short, hard, and effective. He spends just 45 minutes each week on the weights. With that small investment, he has maintained his bodyweight where it was when he was in college (150 lbs.), his body fat at a desirable level (11.9%), and his strength close to where it was when he was 20 years younger.

His most recent breakthrough has been with aerobics. His aerobics journey has followed a pendulum path, from high volume to high intensity to just right for him. He started doing aerobic training in college, but never took it too seriously. He followed the standard prescription of 30 minutes three times per week, staying within his target zone of 65% to 85% of maximum heart rate. He was never tested, so doesn't know how well it worked.

About 20 years later, at 42, he decided to give the Tabata 20-10 protocol a try, and then have his results tested at the Cooper Clinic. He spent just 10 minutes a week on aerobics: a four-minute Tabata protocol twice a week on his stationary bike (with a one-minute warm-up). Amazingly, he did 25 minutes on the CC treadmill test (treadmill incline is increased 1% every minute), which put him in the "excellent" category for his age.

After two more visits to the Cooper Clinic without much improvement, he decided to simply practice the test protocol—applying the specificity principle. That had worked for him as a law student with final exams, so why not here? He bought a treadmill that inclined to 30% so his workouts could precisely mimic the Cooper test. This required more aerobic training time, but he found the test protocol to be friendlier than all-out Tabata intervals. It worked.

With just three 25-minute workouts each week (the first 15 minutes is essentially a long warm-up), he was able to achieve, at age 46, a time of 28:00 minutes, which put him in the top 1% for his age—and in the "superior" category for a 30-year-old.

An added—and very satisfying—bonus has been that he has been able to pass on his knowledge of efficient, high-intensity weight training to his teenage son, Matt, with exceptional results.

Dan can fill in many more of the details:

My "take charge" fitness journey began when I was 15 years old. I was always a good athlete because of strong hand-eye co-

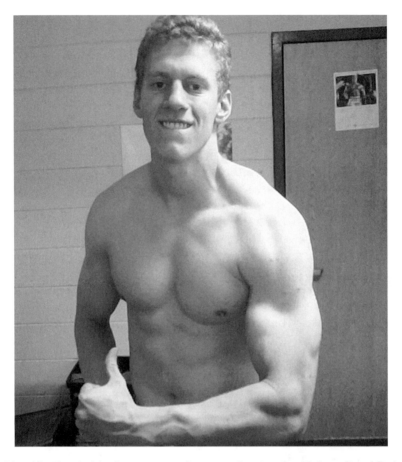

Matt Keating in his dorm room after a workout at the University of Dallas weight room; it shows the results of his dad's coaching and several years of hard and efficient weight training. See page 212 for the before photo. *Photo courtesy of Dan Keating*

ordination, but my ectomorph frame made me naturally skinny and weak. I desperately wanted to get bigger and stronger, and I was willing and eager to put in the work. My problem at that time was that I simply had no idea what I was doing. The muscle magazines of the day were filled with the marathon workouts of champion bodybuilders. So that's where I began my journey: with a lot of sets and probably some overtraining.

Then, shortly after starting college, I began applying the benefits of Clarence's wisdom on training and diet when I read his first book, Ripped. In that book, Clarence explained why he was a fan of high-intensity, low-volume training. The results he achieved were probably the greatest selling point for me of that school of training. From that point on, I approached my training in a much more efficient and productive manner. I was far from huge, but I did put a lot of muscle on my frame from where I began. At 5'10", 150 pounds, I could bench press 200 pounds for eight reps. The extra strength also helped me on the tennis court as a member of the Monmouth College tennis team.

When I entered law school at the University of Chicago, I did not cut back on my training despite the many hours of study that law school required. I remember vividly during first-year final exams how many of my classmates were pulling all-nighters while I continued to work out regularly and get eight hours of sleep each night. Twice during law school I did hydrostatic body fat testing (the "gold standard" for such testing) and achieved body fat levels of 5%, then 4% while maintaining my weight at 150 pounds. Even if I still wasn't huge, I was definitely "ripped."

The focus of my training changed after I graduated from law school, got married, and started having children. As I got into my late 20's and early 30's, I began to appreciate my workouts as much for their overall health benefits as for the cosmetic benefits. I started incorporating aerobics into my workouts, although at that time I was doing the traditional steady state aerobics rather than interval training. I was able to continue lifting weights comparable to what I had lifted in college.

When I reached my early 40's, two new challenges confronted me in my fitness journey. Thanks to information that I learned through Clarence's books and columns, I was able to overcome both of those challenges. My first challenge was that my aging body was starting to protest my continued use of heavy weights. I suffered through a series of injuries, including tendonitis in my elbow and rotator cuff, plus herniated discs in my lower back and my neck. My successful response on this one was what Clarence calls "the effort principle."

The research reported in this book shows that muscle growth depends not necessarily on using the heaviest weights, but rather on pushing your muscles close to failure—even if you use a lighter weight, more reps and slower form to get there. So now the weights I use are lighter than what I once used, but I still get close to failure on each set through a longer time under load. Since changing to this style of lifting, I have maintained my muscle mass but have not had an injury for at least six or seven years.

My second mid-life fitness challenge arose when I discovered from my first visit to the Cooper Clinic at age 42 that I had premature calcium buildup in one of my coronary arteries, which is a significant risk factor for a future heart attack. My response to this news was to start taking aerobics seriously for the first time. On that score, Clarence's extensive reporting of the benefits of interval training convinced me to start using that technique for my aerobic training. On my most recent visit to the Cooper Clinic, at age 48, I was able to achieve a time of 28:16 on the treadmill test. That time put me in the top 1% not only for my age group, but also for the 30-year-old age group. Surprisingly, I was able to achieve that level of fitness by devoting less than an hour each week to aerobic training.

Probably the most gratifying chapter in my "take charge" fitness story has been serving as a trainer for my son Matt, who is now 19. Matt began lifting weights when he was 14. Although Matt is taller than I am, he definitely inherited my ectomorph body type. So, like me, he is a classic "hard gainer." Unlike me in my teenage years, however, Matt did not have to waste any time on unproductive training techniques. By using a training

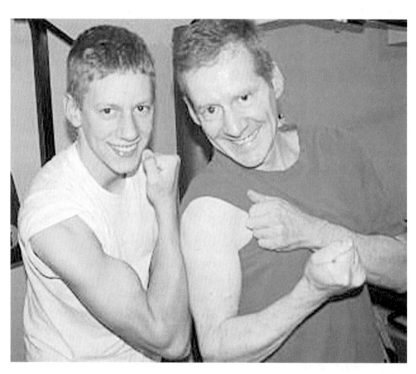

Dan and Matt (14 here) square off in a father-son "arms race." We called it a tie. Five years later, Matt was 19 and about 40 pounds heavier. It was no longer a tie. *Photo courtesy of Dan Keating*

regimen I devised that emphasized high-intensity, single-set, compound exercises, Matt was able to add strength and mass throughout his high school years while devoting somewhere between one and two hours per week to his strength training.

Matt was a three-sport varsity athlete in high school, and his strength training helped his effectiveness in all three sports. In tennis, the extra muscle helped his serve and the overall power of his ground strokes. In basketball, his strength enabled him to lead the league in rebounding for two years in a row despite being relatively short (6'3") for the center position. In football, Matt's lifting enabled him to transform himself from a wide receiver as a freshman to a starting offensive lineman as a senior.

As I reflect on my fitness journey, I am convinced that any of us can "take charge" of our bodies as long as we have two prerequisites: knowledge and discipline. I got my knowledge largely from Clarence and his various publications. I was then able to "pay it forward" by applying that knowledge to Matt and his training. Indeed, I have helped a number of friends get started with their training by teaching them the principles of the research that is so masterfully reported each month on the Ripped *website (cbass.com).*

As we lawyers like to say, however, knowledge is a "necessary but not sufficient" condition for fitness. You still need the will and the discipline to apply the knowledge you gain to your own training. The good news is that there are more options than ever for taking charge of your body in ways that will get you the results you seek. You can choose the path that works best for you, and you need not spend endless hours to achieve your fitness goals.

Inform yourself, chart your own fitness course, and then take the first step (literally and figuratively!) on your new journey.

Wayne Gallasch—World Record Holder at 70

Wayne Gallasch is known for his persistence. Once he sets his mind on a course of action, he is practically unstoppable. He simply won't give up. That makes him a formidable competitor at whatever he undertakes. (As you'll see, I almost crippled myself trying to keep up with him.)

Wayne has traveled the world for almost 50 years, from Australia, filming and later video taping the most important people and events in bodybuilding. His collection is the largest and most wide-ranging in the world. If you want a DVD of an important event or a top bodybuilder, Wayne is the man to contact (gmv.com.au); if he doesn't have it you are probably out of luck.

Not just the historian behind the camera, Wayne has been lifting weights his entire life. He has been both a lifting and physique champion. In 1966, he started competing in power lifting, and in the next five years won the Australian National Championship three times and held the national records in his class for a number of years. In physique competition, he placed second in the Mr. South Australia contest in 1967, and won in 1968.

He retired from competition at the end of 1971, but continued lifting, jogging, and playing squash to stay fit.

Wayne Gallasch and I go way back. He first visited with us in 1983; we have stayed in touch since then. Over the years, Carol and I have become good friends with Wayne and his wife, Tina.

Wayne will take up the story from there:

After visiting you late last year [2002] I received two separate inspirations. One was to move out of my comfort zone with weights and cardio training and secondly to consider the Concept 2 age-based world rankings for indoor rowing as a goal-setting vehicle for self improvement. Although I have been weight training for 40 years, I had never touched a rower apart from an occasional warm-up before a workout.

Due to my constant travel to video tape contests around the world, I was not able to do any serious training till February of this year and that was on the road between contests. I thought I was pretty fit due to years of jogging and some Airdyne training, so imagine my shock when I discovered how hard rowing really is. The first time I attempted 500 meters in February after a couple of days rowing, I couldn't break 2 minutes. My time was a terribly slow 2:03.0.

This really got me interested as I love a challenge. I had some reservations at first that I would not be able to make much progress at my age of 60. In these rankings you will find men who have been rowing for many years and quite a few of them have no doubt been top notch water rowers. By early March, however, I had broken the 2 minute barrier and really felt encouraged to push on.

My training in the gym had also moved out of maintenance mode into "Challenge Yourself mode" with periodization training where you are pushing ahead to harder mini goals, reaching them and moving on again. I had not trained this way before. Tina, my wife, trained along with me. Improvements continued to come for both of us, in the weights we were using and in rowing times.

For example, my squat poundages increased by 60% and similar increases have taken place in the bench press and deadlift. I had not done heavy squats and deadlifts since retiring from power lifting 30 years ago. I thought my days of competition and real improvement were over!

Tina, who is 56, had never done squats and deadlifts. She actually likes both.

It was time to see if our rowing progress was a short term flash in the pan or the real thing. Our home rower didn't have a proper monitor, so we went to a public gym with a Concept 2 rower for another test.

This was in late April, just before I left Australia to cover some bodybuilding events in Europe, where I am now. Imagine our joint excitement: My 500 meter time improved by 11 seconds, and Tina improved by 9 seconds.

This really fired me up for more improvement. I managed to find a gym in Essen, Germany, and get in several good workouts. They didn't have a rower, but plenty of weights. Now I am in England and fortunately found a gym in Cambridge with 5 Concept 2 rowers. Over the last 2 weeks I have been training hard, lots of Tabata intervals on the rower. This is my last day at this gym before moving on to some new unknown gym up in the north of England. So it is now rowing D-Day, 1 week before my 61st birthday.

Success!

I'm very pleased to be able to post online a 500 meter time of 1:41.9. This is an improvement of 4.6 seconds on my effort one month ago and ranks me (temporarily) #1 in the Concept 2 World Rankings as a lightweight, or 5th overall in my age group.

All this goes to prove that whatever your age, you can make substantial and steady improvement. It may not be that you will bench press more than you did when you were 25. But there are many different areas you can explore to find ways of self improvement both in rowing times, or in weight used, or reps achieved with different weights. The possibilities are endless. I plan to go on improving in different areas for as long as I can get into the gym. Whatever I achieve I always feel I can beat it next time! This sort of competition gets the best out of yourself and, as you say, you don't have to be # 1 in the world rankings to be a winner.

Tina has also gone up remarkably well in training poundages

and in her rowing times, where she is presently #2 in Australia in her class.

Thanks Clarence for the motivation and inspiration. We both have a new perspective on training, on diet and on life. We plan to train hard and smart and preferably in a stable environment, not always while living out of a suitcase!

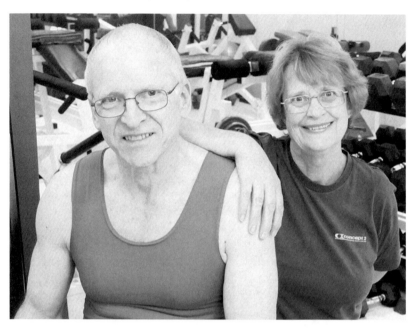

Wayne and Tina are a team to be reckoned with. Tina not only provides support, she lifts and rows with Wayne. An excellent coach, she keeps him "on plan" during workouts and competition.

Photo courtesy of Wayne and Tina Gallasch

* * *

As noted earlier, Wayne is a dogged competitor. He was just getting started.

On June 4, 2003, a few days after writing the above letter, Wayne served notice that he would not easily relinquish his first place ranking. Making another quantum leap forward in his meteoric rowing career, he posted a 500-meter time of 1:38.3. He was now more than 8 seconds ahead of the second-place time and not far from the best time posted the previous season. He set his sight on 1:35 before Christmas.

In less than six months, Wayne had gone from a beginner to first in the world for his age and weight. As it turned out, he really was just getting started.

He finished the season in first place, with a phenomenal time of 1:34.1, 3.5 seconds ahead of the second place finisher. (I almost crippled myself trying to keep up with my acolyte—and now nemesis—finishing in 5th place with a time of 1:38.6.)

Emboldened by his early success at 500 meters, Wayne decided to try his hand at the Olympic 2000 meter distance—at the British Indoor Rowing Championship (BIRC). (Wayne learned of the event while planning his travel schedule for taping the Mr. Universe contest in London.)

The BIRC is the biggest indoor rowing event in the world! Rowers compete from many different countries, including the USA. Wayne would be competing along with 4000 other rowers in Britain's biggest-ever participatory indoor sports event.

With a little over three months of preparation, Wayne placed a very respectable 6th in his age and weight category with a time of 7 minutes and 30 seconds, beating his previous best by 10 seconds. It was like playing tennis at Wimbledon—and doing well your first time out. (You'll find many more details on Wayne's BIRC experience at cbass.com.)

The next year, Wayne improved his 500 meter time to 1:33.2, but dropped back to second place in the C2 world ranking. The first place time was a daunting 1:29.9. Wayne's time was remarkable, but his rate of improvement had slowed dramatically.

*   *   *

After his astounding rise in indoor rowing competition, Wayne settled back into training for fitness. He kept rowing, but didn't compete again until 2012, when he came roaring back. He wanted to leave his mark in the 60-69 age category—and burst onto the scene in the 70-79 age category. Once again, he was not to be denied.

Wayne and I had established a tradition of training together at least once a year. So I was able to observe his condition during his hiatus from competition. He kept training, but gained weight and let his condition slip from where it was when he was rowing competitively. That changed when he turned 69—and how.

Wayne won four Gold Medals in indoor rowing at the 2012 New Zealand Masters Games. Twelve countries competed, including the USA. Wayne cleaned up in the 65-69 age category, lightweight class, winning at 2000m, 1000m, 500m, and 300m—all on the same day. It was an amazing performance.

Wayne visited with us soon after his New Zealand sweep. Preparing for that competition had him looking terrific. He was about 10 pounds lighter than when we saw him last and had leaned out all over his body. He had muscle from head to toe that few men half his age can match. A combination of careful eating, weight training, and rowing had done wonderful things for him. (Unfortunately, it couldn't do anything about his gray hair—but at least he had hair.)

I expected him to be the best in the world at 500 meters when he moved into the 70-79 age category. He met my expectations and more.

A few days *before* turning 70, on May 30, 2012, he broke his own 500 meter Australian record in the men's 60-69 lightweight class with a time of 1:33.9, 0.6 faster than his old record. Twelve days after turning 70, he smashed the 500 meter world record for lightweight men 70 to 79—by 4.2 seconds. His time was 1:34.2. The old world record was held by Dean Smith of the USA, set 7 years previously.

Wayne now has his eye on Roger Bangay's 1000m age-group record. Great Britain's Bangay holds the world records from 1000m to marathon distance (42,195m). He won the 2012 world championship in the very competitive 2000m distance, having prevailed at the 31st annual Crash-B Sprints held in Boston. Bangay is a certified legend. He and Wayne are good friends; Bangay is respected around the world and Wayne is the new guy on the 70-to-79 block. Breaking one of Bangay's records would be an epic achievement. If anyone can do it, Wayne can.

Postscript

My Training Routine, In Brief

Bits and pieces of my training routine are scattered throughout this book. That doesn't mean that what I do is the best choice; I make no such claim. The key is to exercise regularly—in a way that works for you; that's what I do. The purpose of this book is to help you find the most effective way—for you. That's what taking charge is about. I wouldn't blindly follow anyone else's routine, and I don't expect anyone to follow mine.

In *Ripped 2*, my second book, I quoted the following maxim with approval: "Surely the quickest path to disillusionment is the one blazed by someone else." That was 30 years ago—and I stand by it.

Nevertheless, I know that readers want to know what I do; one of the most frequently asked questions about our books is, "Does it include Clarence's training routine?"

With that preface, here's a brief overview of what I do day to day. (Parenthetical references to the chapter covering the particular component are also included.)

I'll do my best to keep it simple, but the many moving parts tend to cloud the picture. Focus on the grand plan and you'll see that the routine is more transparent than most.

I begin most days with my *Morning Motion* wake-up routine before breakfast and take short walks (~10 minutes) at convenient times during the day. I also make it a point to get up and move around periodically when working at the computer or my desk. (See Chapter 7: Too Much Sitting)

Walking is the only moderate-to-easy steady state exercise I do.

I work out three days a week (Sunday, Wednesday, and Saturday) alternating hard and easy workouts. For example, if Sunday is a hard day one week, it's easy the next week. The result is two hard days one week and two easy days the next week.

Weekly workouts are balanced, half strength and half aerobics. Sunday is primarily strength training and Saturday is primarily aerobic training. Wednesday is a combination of strength and aerobics. (See Chapter 4: The Aerobic-Strength Alliance)

Strength movements are primarily multi-joint (leg press, bent row, bench press, and shoulder press, for example); this keeps workouts short and efficient. Aerobic sessions are mostly intervals, with some single sprints. (See Chapter 3: The Rise of Intervals) Training time is usually an hour or less. Strength workouts tend to be longer and aerobic sessions shorter.

In both strength and aerobic training, my focus is on effort. I try to improve from week to week. I have a plan for every workout. When I hit a sticking point, weights or aerobics, I pull back and start up again. (See Chapter 2: Forget Heavy, Think Effort)

The Sunday hard day and easy day strength workouts differ in more than intensity. The hard day is entirely weight training, while the easy day includes bodyweight movements (push-ups, chin-ups, back extensions, and hip curls, for example). In addition, the easy day ends with 10 minutes of intervals (Lifecycle or Schwinn Airdyne). (See Chapter 4: The Aerobic-Strength Alliance)

As noted, Wednesday is a combination of strength and aerobic training. Strength training is primarily upper body, while aerobic training alternates between lower body (Lifecycle) and whole body (Airdyne). As before, I alternate hard days and easy days.

Finally, Saturday is my shortest, hardest—and newest—workout. It's entirely devoted to short intervals (work periods one minute or less) or single sprints from 250 meters to 1000 meters, combining the Concept 2 Rower and the Concept 2 Ski Erg.

The Concept 2 Rower is not new; I've been using and writing about it since the publication of *Lean For Life* in 1989. What is

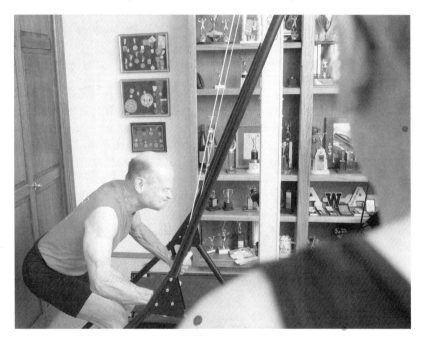

This photo by Laszlo shows me near the bottom of the downward pull on the C2 Ski Erg. I made a 500-meter PR during the photo shoot for this book; this shows me near the end. Wayne Gallasch was there to observe; he's on the right.

new is the Ski Erg, which was introduced by Concept 2 in 2009. We purchased ours early in 2012.

Concept 2 touts the similarity of the motion to cross-country skiing, which produces some of the fittest athletes in the world. That's intriguing, but alone probably wouldn't have persuaded me to buy one. What caught my attention is that the Ski Erg complements the Rower. The Rower extends the body, while the Ski Erg flexes the body. Put the two together and you have a combo that trains practically the whole body.

The icing on the cake is the superb performance monitor that comes on both the rower and the Ski Erg. The monitor assesses your pace on every pull or stroke, while timing, counting, and recalling every interval or sprint. It's perfect for tracking progress—down to the fraction of a second. It also allows you to compete on both machines with others your age and weight around the world. (I compete at 500 meters and 1000 meters.)

I do intervals or sprints on both machines back to back. I start with the rower one Saturday and with the Ski Erg the next. (I don't rush from machine to machine; I rest as long as I need.) That's the Saturday workout. I can do any sprint distance or work/rest ratio I want. I try to improve workout to workout on both machines, changing distance or work/rest ratio from week to week and backing off when I hit a sticking point. (See again Chapter 3: The Rise of Intervals)

It works beautifully. The entire workout takes well short of an hour, including warm-up and cool-down. I eat after the workout and then lie down for about an hour. It's a perfect fit for Saturday, when I have more time to devote to training. (To learn more about both units, visit www.concept2.com.)

One more very important point: In keeping with the latest research, I emphasize intensity over volume. Intensity becomes more important with age. If you take only one point away from my routine, that would be the one. (See Chapter 6: Exercise and Aging)

That's it. That's my current training routine. It works for me and may give you some ideas you can put to work in your own routine.

Good training to you all!

Acknowledgments

I am blessed with a long "thank you" list, the longest in my writing career.

This book is dedicated to Carole Wright and Dr. Ralph Carpinelli. Carole has been in our corner since before we knew she was there. She worked for the people who assembled our first book in 1980 and noticed that some of the photos were not cropped properly. Without telling us or anyone else, she came in on her own time and "fixed" them. She has been an important member of our team ever since, placing the words and photos in our books and ads for over 30 years.

Dr. Carpinelli politely declined our request for a photo to appear in this book. He is very private in his personal life, but unflinching in his research. His meticulous analysis of the "heavier is better" approach to resistance training inspired this book. He also made helpful suggestions on parts of our manuscript.

Pat Berrett has been photographing me for over 20 years. He has focused on physique and exercise photos. That's what we've asked him to do and he has done it extremely well. Photos are a bodybuilder's stock and trade. Pat's camera expertise has allowed me to showcase my results—very important for a bodybuilder who writes extensively about his diet and training. To have him available locally has been a godsend.

Laszlo Bencze has brought a new perspective to our photos. A lifetime strength trainer, he travels the world taking photos for mining companies, pharmaceutical companies, you name it. This unique combination has brought a new look and feel to the photos in our last book and this book. He lived with us for a week both times and constantly came up with new ways to present our lifestyle to the public. The very different cover photo on this book is an example.

Richard Winett is my oldest friend in the academic world; we've been corresponding regularly for almost 30 years. Like Laszlo, Richard has been training with weights his entire adult life. Like me, he has included some form of aerobic exercise in his routine for many years. He informed me about the Schwinn Airdyne and the Tabata Protocol. A professor of psychology, he alerted me to many psychological concepts relating to health and fitness, including *Flow*. He also introduced me to the work of Ralph Carpinelli and Stuart Phillips. Where would I be without Dick Winett?

Professor Stuart Philips has freely given of his time to help me understand the emerging connection between strength and endurance exercise. A query to Dr. Philips gets a quick and complete response.

Terry Todd and I have known each other since our early lifting years; he claims to be younger than me, but the truth is that I am only a day or two older. We have come to know each other better in recent years. He told Dr. Waneen Spirduso, his colleague at the University of Texas (Austin), about me when she was looking for an older bodybuilder to include in the second edition of her landmark text *Physical Dimensions of Aging*. Todd also displayed a series of my photos in the opening exhibit of the Joe and Betty Weider Museum at the Stark Center for Physical Culture and Sports. (Terry and his wife Jan are co-directors of the Stark Center.) While Terry has not been directly involved in this book, he has encouraged and helped me in many ways. For example, he alerted me to *Bending the Aging Curve*, the book by Professor Joseph Signorile.

Dr. Signorile reviewed the first seven chapters of our manuscript and made a number of useful suggestions. He is a master of commenting without seeming to criticize. "Dr. Sig," his students complain, "you never give us any absolute answers." That's because "over the years everything that we present as an *absolute* changes," he returns. I generally don't take well to "suggestions," but the Signorile version goes down smoothly.

Wade Smith, an orthopedic trauma surgeon and professor at the University of Colorado School of Medicine (and a former world record holder in speed skating), has also been very supportive of our efforts in recent years, especially so regarding this book.

Dan Keating, a professor of law and one of our "Take Charge People," is the only outside person to review our entire manuscript. He has an uncanny eye for typos and an amazing ability to "connect the dots." Dan "gets it" like no one else.

Carl Miller is my oldest friend in weightlifting. We competed against one another in the Teenage National Championship. Carl went on to become the United States Weightlifting Coach at the Montreal Olympic Games and now operates a highly regarded fitness center in Santa Fe, New Mexico. Carl is the quintessential coach and a friend like no other.

I also want to acknowledge the many people who send me column topics each month. They know who they are. Without them a book like this would not be possible. A tip of the hat to each and every one of them.

Finally, my wife Carol has been a partner in all of our books.

In this book, however, she really got down in the weeds. I wrote the first draft of each chapter and then she got out her editing pencil and went to work. We kept going back and forth until we were both satisfied. It hasn't always been pretty or fun, but working together we believe we have produced a reader friendly and useful book.

Carol is the love of my life. She also makes our train run on time. Without her it's unlikely that you would be reading this.